PRAISE FOR F~~IGHT LIKE~~

"RIP Luke. The impact you made in my life will never be forgotten. #TeamLuke."

– Patrick Mahomes,
Quarterback for the Kansas City Chiefs

"If you want to be inspired you MUST read this book by Tim Siegel about his son Luke. In 2015 his son was seriously injured in a golf cart accident. Luke suffered a brain injury that was life-changing for his family. The love demonstrated by his dad in the seven years that Luke fought for his life captivated so many nationally. On August 19, 2021, Luke lost his life but will live on forever as he made such an impact on so many in the 15 years he lived. The dedication by his dad to Team Luke and to helping others dealing with brain injuries will continue to impact so many. This book is about a father's love for his son and in writing it, his son's life will live on through TEAM LUKE. In short, it's "AWESOME BABY," with a capital A!"

– Dick Vitale,
American Sportscaster

"Getting to know Luke Siegel was an absolute honor and one that I will cherish forever. Luke is a massive inspiration to me and countless others. At the same time, his story is a stark reminder about how precious life can be. I simply cannot imagine the grief the Siegel family is going through, but I know the work Luke's father, Tim, is doing with Team Luke Hope for Minds, is truly God's work and it will always keep Luke's legacy going. I consider myself so lucky to have known Luke and am a proud supporter of the amazing foundation in his name."

– **John Isner,**
Professional Tennis Player

"As an All-American, professional, and D-1 college tennis coach, Tim Siegel knows about being down a set and fighting back. But his prolific athletic career could not prepare him for the setbacks he suffered in life. Living through the pain of losing his son, not once but twice, has required Tim to find a new grip to pull him through. Now in this new part of his story, he extends that hand back to us."

– **Chuck Angel,**
Pastor at Turning Point Community Church

FIGHT LIKE LUKE

TRANSFORMING GRIEF INTO LOVE, STRENGTH, AND FAITH

J Siegel

TIM SIEGEL

Luke 8:39

ISBN 13: 978-1-954020-40-5 (Paperback)
ISBN 13: 978-1-954020-41-2 (Ebook)

Library of Congress Cataloging-in-Publication Data
Names: Siegel, Tim, author.
Title: Fight Like Luke / Tim Siegel
Description: First Edition | Texas: Per Capita Publishing (2022)
Identifiers: LCCN 2022916016 (print)

First Edition

ALL AUTHOR'S PROCEEDS OF *FIGHT LIKE LUKE*
WILL GO TO TEAM LUKE HOPE FOR MINDS.

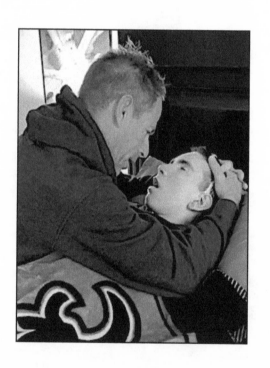

This book is dedicated to Luke.
My boy, my hero, and my inspiration.
And to my family.
Without you, I wouldn't be able to put one
foot in front of the other.

TABLE OF CONTENTS

FOREWORD

Jesus answered, I am the way, and the truth, and the life. No
one comes to the Father except through me.
— John 14:6

I am a man of faith. Everything I do as a husband, a father,
and a football player is always with God in my heart and
in my soul.

I'm a very blessed man. My beautiful wife Tamela means
the world to me; she is my rock and an amazing mom to our
four children. I love football, but the love I have for my Lord
and Savior and for my family is unmatched.

God has allowed me to play this wonderful game of
football for many years. I played football for Arkansas State
where I found trouble along the way, and eventually God
became my way and prepared me for life in the NFL. Football has taught me many things: leadership, discipline, the
highs and lows of victories and losses, and the opportunity

to work together as a team.

I played for the New York Jets and the Cleveland Browns before joining the New Orleans Saints for the 2018 season. I thank God every day that I get to play linebacker for this first-class organization, and for the best fans in the NFL.

I'm honored to be able to give back to the community of New Orleans. This is a priority of mine, as well as many of my teammates.

In June 2022, we announced my vision of the Devoted Dreamers Academy, a school that will be designed to serve New Orleans youth through sports, academics, and mentorship. Tamela and I began the Devoted Dreamers Foundation in 2013, which equips the next generation of leaders with tools to be successful spiritually, mentally, and physically. I will continue to do my best to impact and inspire kids in Louisiana, Mississippi, and all over the region.

But sometimes I am the one inspired and impacted by kids.

On November 10, 2019, the Saints were about to host our big rival, the Atlanta Falcons. Our warm-up had just ended, and the team was headed back to the locker room, when I noticed a young boy in a wheelchair.

I felt at that very moment God calling me to pray over him. I leaned over the boy and prayed to God to restore him and I told that precious little boy that "it's in God's hands." (I later found out that Tim Siegel had written a book called *It's in God's Hands* in 2019.)

That boy was Luke Siegel. His father reached out to me to come to Lubbock, Texas for a fundraiser for Team Luke

Hope for Minds, which is a nonprofit that supports children after brain injury. Tim had started this nonprofit because Luke had suffered a brain injury in 2015.

Tim's love and devotion for Luke has inspired me to be a better father. And Luke's fight will forever have an impact on my life.

In May 2022, I had the incredible honor of speaking in Lubbock, Texas, in front of 500 of the friendliest, most supportive people I've ever been around. The event raised money for children with brain injuries and was an evening I will never forget.

Luke's favorite team was the Saints, and I'm honored to play for his team. He has inspired my family and the entire New Orleans Saints organization.

I will fight like Luke every play for the rest of my NFL career.

And we know that all that happens to us is working for our good if we love God and are fitting into his plans.
— Romans 8:28

– **Demario Davis**
New Orleans Saints

PROLOGUE

I have always loved coaching, but I loved being with my family more. I wanted to be home for my children; to be with my wife, Jenny, my three girls, and my son. After the tremendous honor of coaching, teaching, and impacting young men for 23 years, it was finally time for me to resign as the men's tennis coach at Texas Tech University.

My dream as long as I can remember was to play professional tennis. That dream came true through a lot of hard work. Playing Wimbledon, the US Open, and all the big tournaments was a thrill . . . as well as playing against some of the biggest names in our sport. John McEnroe, Stefan Edberg, Ivan Lendl, and Yannick Noah were just a few of the names I faced on the other side of the net.

But my ultimate dream, my long-term dream, was to

be a father. I wanted to be a girl dad, and I wanted to have a son.

By the time I retired, my daughter Alex was 23 years old and was ready to be a full-time nurse. Kate was 12, Ellie 10, and Luke was nine. All three played sports, and God knows I never wanted to miss a practice or game.

I resolved to make a greater impact on middle school and high school tennis players. Yes, I would teach them and coach them, but I wanted to inspire them and teach them about life. On July 8, 2015, I resigned as the Head Men's Tennis Coach at Texas Tech, and two days later I was named the tennis coach at Laura Bush Middle School and the head coach at Lubbock Cooper High School.

As I drove home that afternoon, there was no doubt who was going to greet me at the front door. Sure enough, Luke came outside ready to throw the football. Without hesitation I told Luke that I had just resigned from Texas Tech. He looked at me with uncertainty and said, "So now we're gonna have to sit in the stands with those people?" My office overlooked the Texas Tech football field and according to Luke, that was the best perk of my job. I then looked into his beautiful blue eyes and gave him some good news: "But now we can go to the Rangers spring training games." He smiled. And then he smiled some more when I said that we would go to more Saints and Texas Rangers games.

Luke had such a sweet soul. He loved being with his friends, and whatever they wanted to do, he was happy to oblige. One of the nicest things anyone ever said about Luke came from a mom whose son was in Luke's third grade class.

She said that Luke had a way of making each one of his friends feel like they were his best friend.

He loved sports. I mean he really, really loved sports. His passion was baseball. His goal was to be the best second baseman in the world. He knew that wouldn't happen without a strong work ethic, and Luke loved to practice. We never missed a day of playing catch, working on groundballs, or throwing the football. In the backyard we worked on his arm and his glove, and in the front yard, I was Drew Brees throwing to Darren Sproles and Marques Colston. Luke loved Drew Brees. He was Luke's hero.

I'm from New Orleans and it was against the law to be just a casual fan of the Saints. Our fans are as ardent as any fan base in the NFL. Luke quickly bought in to being a passionate fan and may have even gone overboard! When they lost it was a heartbreaker; we were both unapproachable. I vividly remember Luke looking down while sitting on the couch as the Cleveland Browns kicked the game winner against the Saints, and when he and Jenny were driving to get ice cream with the radio on as they heard that the Atlanta Falcons had just defeated the New Orleans Saints on a last-second field goal. He was in the back seat with tears rolling down his cheek and refused to talk to his mom.

Luke knew every player and all the stars from every team. He also knew the type of player I liked: hard-nosed, blue-collar, great teammate, maximum effort, and coachable.

Luke and I enjoyed three games together in the Superdome and a memorable one in Dallas as the Saints won on a last-second field goal. Just before the kick I held Luke's hand for good luck. That was a very special moment for father and son.

My favorite Saints story shows Luke's love for our team and his remarkable maturity for a young fan. I had just finished practice with my tennis team when I looked at my phone. I immediately called Luke with the news that the Saints traded tight end Jimmy Graham. There was silence on the other end. Luke was crying as I explained why the Saints made the trade.

That evening Luke came up to me at the kitchen table, and these words came out of his mouth: "Dad, I'm beginning to understand why we made this trade. We now have a better center, and a first-round draft pick, which will help our defense." I just had to hug him. Proud dad moment.

The one thing I loved to do was watch my kids compete, in practice and in games. All four of them knew I was proud of them if their effort was good: Alex in tennis, Kate in basketball and volleyball, Ellie in volleyball and competitive cheer, and Luke in baseball and flag football.

Sports were a big part of our family, but my absolute favorite time of the week was when I sat with Kate, Ellie, and Luke at their lunch. Once a week, every week, and one at a time. The best two hours of the week.

Our evenings consisted of shooting baskets, throwing the ball, homework, and watching sports on TV. Most nights Jenny would ask me to put Luke to bed. As soon as we got into his room, we smiled at each other, and I turned a ball game on. At least we were in bed!

Life was good. With my job change, a new challenge was in front of me, and I was looking forward to it. Best of all, I would be home more. No more long road trips recruiting all over the world, and no more sleepless nights agonizing over a heartbreaking loss.

This new chapter of life was just beginning, and I had a timeframe. My goal was to coach middle school and high school for nine years, until Luke graduated. Just a few days after I resigned from Texas Tech, Luke and I went to a park to play tennis, which he had recently showed an interest in playing. I'll never forget what he said as we were picking up the balls:

"Dad, I can't wait for you to help me improve my tennis, so one day I can play for you."

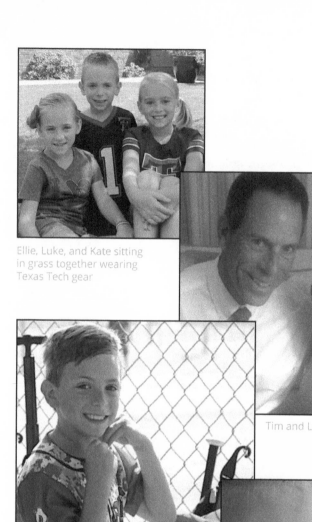

Ellie, Luke, and Kate sitting in grass together wearing Texas Tech gear

Tim and Luke

Luke at a baseball game

Luke with "WHO DAT" written with face paint

01

JULY 28, 2015

"Be thankful for today, because in one moment,
your entire life could change."
— Unknown[1]

I was coaching at Cooper High School on a hot summer day when my cell phone rang. I looked around at all six courts full of enthusiastic tennis players and thought that this new experience was exactly what I needed. Coaching high school kids who wanted to be motivated and inspired was in my blood. I had been feeding balls on court number two when my phone rang. "Luke has been in a golf cart accident."

I raced to the scene of the accident, where a fireman promptly yelled at me to get to the hospital. The ambulance had just left when I arrived, and to my surprise there was a helicopter hovering above us. I remember wondering: Why didn't they take Luke in the helicopter instead of an ambulance, when there was a big field right next to the scene of the accident? Just one of many questions that are still unanswered.

My journey to the hospital was a blur. Just a few minutes

after meeting Jenny at the hospital, we were approached by a doctor. As we were still reeling from what had happened, he took us into a small room and broke the news—news that continues to haunt me.

"The golf cart landed on top of Luke. He suffered head and chest trauma, and he was in cardiac arrest for seven minutes."

Suddenly my hands went numb. My breathing was getting faster. I leaned against the wall yelling, "No, no, no!"

I couldn't feel my face or my hands. I vaguely remember telling my daughter Alex to grab my phone and let a few people know what had just happened. I was panicking. Cardiac arrest? No, this can't be real. Just then a nurse raised her voice and said, "Luke needs you to be strong." Those words were true, but they didn't diminish my anxiety. I could barely breathe. I remember hearing someone tell me to take deep breaths. Next thing I knew, there was an oxygen mask in my face. The fact that Jenny is a nurse practitioner was both a good thing and a bad thing. The good thing was that she understood what the doctors were saying—and the bad thing was that she knew what the doctors were saying.

Every time a doctor or nurse would discuss with us Luke's condition, I would immediately turn to Jenny, and her reaction said it all. One question she asked them in particular concerned me: "Why was Luke anoxic if he spoke at the scene?" The first responders at the scene of the accident came to visit Luke just a few hours after he arrived at the hospital. One of them said that Luke answered two questions just minutes after the accident. "Luke, do you play baseball?" "Are you any good?" He had answered yes to both. When I heard this my heart began to explode out of my chest. He spoke, but now he is in an induced coma.

The first few nights were touch and go. Luke was battling chest and head trauma—an awfully dangerous combination.

Luke made it through the first six days, and on day seven, I noticed the numbers indicating Luke's brain pressure was rising. The doctors had told me that anything under 20 was good.

I began to panic as the numbers climbed above 25. Shortly after, the surgeon came in and performed three major surgeries: cranioplasty, craniectomy, and duraplasty. Cranioplasty is a surgical operation to repair cranial defects and is performed by filling the defective area with a range of materials, usually a bone piece from the patient. A craniectomy is a type of surgery to remove a portion of the skull to help relieve pressure on the brain. A duraplasty is a reconstructive operation on the open dura matter that involves a primary closure with another soft tissue material.

An hour later, Luke was taken to the operating room for yet another operation intended to relieve the brain pressure. It didn't work either, and now I was more than worried—I was petrified.

Later that night, Luke was taken back for a third operation. Two hours later they wheeled him back to his room in the ICU. I asked the doctor if this didn't work, what he would try next. He responded, "There is nothing else I can do. I'm out of options. It's in God's hands."

My heart was in my chest as they hooked everything back into his room. Everything was now turned on. I could barely look; I was so nervous. Slowly the numbers rose to 15, 20, 25, and just as I felt that familiar panic settle in at the prospect of yet another surgery, the numbers began to drop to normal levels. My knees gave out and I sat down on the floor of the lobby trying to catch my breath. This crisis was averted . . . but what could possibly happen next?

The doctor seemed pleased at the turn of brain pressure, but then he said something I did not expect. "I still don't know if Luke is brain dead." Brain dead? How can you not know? Luke went through over eight hours of surgeries, and we still didn't have an answer. I took a deep breath and from that point forward I exhibited more patience than I ever thought possible. We would find out soon enough, so in the meantime, I prayed and prayed and prayed.

The next afternoon, an intensivist walked into Luke's room and asked us if he liked music. Next to sports, music was his favorite passion, all kinds of music. Hearing this, the doctor pulled out his ukulele from its case. He began playing the song, "Stand by Me." I stood next to Luke and watched and listened to those very poignant words. We were standing by Luke, and so was God.

After a while of looking back and forth from Luke and the monitor, I suddenly saw wavy lines—lines that indicated brain activity. I stayed long enough to make sure it wasn't a fluke, that the other people in the room had seen it too, before I thanked God and the doctor and ran downstairs. A good friend was just outside, and I asked him if we could throw the football. I needed to release all my built-up emotions over the last eight days. I knew the battle was just beginning, and Luke would need me to be levelheaded, present, and competent. I would shake it off and get back to it.

Over the next 36 days, Luke underwent multiple surgeries. Each time, my little fighter pulled through.

Jenny spent most of her time in Luke's room. I did the opposite. Those first few weeks we had hundreds of visitors. Friends, family, and people I didn't know came at all hours of the day. I found out later that there were signs in front of restaurants that said, "Pray for Luke," and multiple stories on the news updating our community on Luke's progress. Jenny was comfortable staying in Luke's room. I would visit in his room, but for me, talking to those visitors in the waiting area seemed to calm my nerves. Time went by faster and most of the time I was talking but not even aware of what I was saying. My mind was going a hundred miles an hour. In the early mornings, I paced the halls praying and said the same thing over and over: "Luke, you're my boy." Every time I said that to Luke prior to the accident, he would nod his head and say, "Sure, Dad." Saying this in the hospital gave me strength. God knows I needed it.

On September 10, 2015, Luke and Jenny were airlifted to Cook Children's Hospital in Fort Worth; he was airlifted due to his condition. I was so worried about them both. Jenny was on antianxiety medication due to everything going on, and my boy needed something that they couldn't provide at our local hospital. As the plane left the ground, my brave face gave way and I collapsed sobbing, punching the ground. This was a necessary change, but the stress had us all on a very thin tightrope.

Cook Children's Hospital is without question the best hospital I have ever seen. The staff were immediately friendly, knowledgeable, and did a wonderful job with the entire family. With the change in scenery came a new, improved attitude; I was confident that Luke would improve at Cook, that he was in good hands.

But five days after arriving, Jenny and I had a life-changing meeting in a conference room with a social worker, therapists, nurses, and our neurologist. They discussed their plan for Luke, which up until now was up in the air for us because we were dealing with the day-to-day aspects of Luke's recovery. They mentioned the therapies he would have each day. I wondered how he would even do anything in therapy. Was he in good enough condition to actually attempt PT, OT, or speech, I asked? They agreed that it might take time but eventually he would be able to participate in the therapies to an extent. Jenny and I sat in silence but felt optimistic that this team would get the most out of Luke. The last person to speak was the neurologist. "I hate to be the bearer of bad news, but Luke's brain is globally damaged. Based on his MRI, Luke will never use his limbs, will never use his voice, and should never open his eyes." This rocked us to our core. Not that we thought Luke would come out on the other side unscathed, but it being said so bluntly was shocking and upsetting.

One by one, they all walked out of the room in silence.

Jenny was sobbing, but I only had one thing on my mind. Before the neurologist left the room, I asked him one last question: "Have you ever seen a patient improve with an MRI this grim?" He nodded, and that was all I needed to see. There is always hope, no matter how small.

At Cook Children's we were supposed to do rehab, PT, OT, and speech. But very rarely did Luke get through a session without elevated blood pressure, spiking heart rate, and vomiting. He needed at least one of us to be there with him every day, helping and encouraging him. Jenny and I decided that she would stay with Luke in Fort Worth while I took care of the girls back in Lubbock and coached the students of Cooper High and Laura Bush Middle School.

Every Tuesday, I drove the 4.5 hours to Cook Children's, spent five hours with Jenny and Luke, then drove back to Lubbock. Occasionally, I had a friend drive with me so I could rest. On Friday afternoon, I took the girls with me and stayed in Fort Worth until Sunday afternoon.

That first month was incredibly hard on Jenny. Her anxiety, her lack of sleep, and Luke's condition took a massive toll on her. A couple of weeks after arriving at Cook, I walked into the hospital with Kate and Ellie, only to be stopped by a nurse. "Your wife is in the ER," she said as we rushed to where she was being kept. Jenny had had such a severe panic attack that she couldn't swallow and struggled to breathe. I couldn't let her take on this emotional toll anymore, at least not for a while.

I took over for Jenny in Fort Worth so she could be with the girls for Halloween. She was to relieve me in two days, but I received a call that she had suffered another panic attack. Soon after hearing this, I called Jenny and insisted that she stay home with the girls to get some rest.

That night I learned how to change a trach. I wrote notes on every medicine that Luke was given. I threw myself into absolutely everything that Luke was experiencing. My biggest issue was the monitors. Once again, I stared at them all day and all night. Every time something was elevated, so too was my heart rate.

Sleeping in Luke's room was optional. I was lucky to get two to three hours a night, but I didn't care about sleep. My only thoughts were to take care of my boy.

In early November, we were told that Luke wasn't making enough progress, and we would have to go home soon. I asked if we could wait until the end of the month. I didn't want to leave. I pleaded for them to let us stay. I had faith that he would soon give us a sign that he was in there, and that he was able to understand.

The Friday before Thanksgiving was a day I'll never forget. He made a sound, and then another, then the amazing nurses on the fourth floor came running into his room. This had been the first time he made a sound in three months. I was on cloud nine. My boy made a sound! I hugged every nurse that came into his room. Everyone was so excited, and I was one proud dad.

But eventually Luke's progress stalled. He continued to make sounds, but that was it. No improvement in PT, OT, or speech, and he was unable to respond to any commands. Everyone insisted that Luke would improve at home. And that would be so much better for our family.

January 6, 2016, five months after Luke's accident, we were finally home. A new life was going to begin for Luke and for our entire family. We'd all have to adjust to a different life for Luke, the girls, and Jenny and me. Kate and Ellie were unsure how to be around Luke. What to say? What not to say? Jenny and I had to learn a new schedule. When to feed Luke, when to give meds, and when to give Luke the rest he needed. We also had to figure out our new schedule. I did my best to coach tennis a couple hours a day while Jenny sat with Luke, then I relieved her so she could work or run errands and spend time with the girls. Our girls had their school activities and we figured out how to tag-team attending their events and taking care of Luke.

A few days later Luke began his therapy routine. The therapists had heard about Luke and were so eager to help him in his recovery. I did not want to miss one session; I wanted to learn everything. The father in me, the coach in me, felt the need to encourage, push, and motivate Luke the best I could.

From therapies, to feeds, to meds . . . I tried to learn what he needed. There were plenty of frightening moments early on, but Jenny was patient with my questions and struggles in the process.

The first few months were an incredible adjustment for everyone. Alex used her nursing skills to take care of her brother. Kate and Ellie were dealing with so much—their brother wasn't the same and neither were they. Friends and teachers always asked them how Luke was doing, but no one asked how they were doing. Their relationship with their brother had rapidly deteriorated and they felt untethered to him and the rest of the family. I remember one of my girls saying, "Dad, I don't even know if Luke knows who we are." Hearing that absolutely crushed me. They were so close, and now they wondered if he even knew who they were. I asked them to talk to Luke, and to be patient. I made sure to convince them that Luke knew who they were. We talked about telling Luke stories, and games that we had watched. Maybe, just maybe, this would ignite something in Luke.

The challenges the first year of therapy were many. Throwing up was a common occurrence as well as elevated blood pressure and heart rate levels. But he never stopped fighting.

In order to provide Luke with the needed expertise and help necessary, we welcomed Astrid into our home as our night nurse. She was with Luke three to four nights a week and quickly became part of our family, bearing witness to our hardest and most miraculous moments.

I wanted to find ways to improve our communications. Initially I would ask Luke to blink if it was a yes answer, for example, "Luke, do you know how much I love you?" He would blink, but I wasn't certain if he blinked to my command or if he was simply blinking because he needed to. I constantly talked to Luke before, during, and after therapies to see if I could connect in a new or different way.

Then something magical happened. The Saints were about to play the Denver Broncos on TV in November of 2016. I was walking Luke in the wheelchair around the living room when I stopped to ask him a question. "Luke, can you move your tongue if you think the Saints are going to beat the Broncos?"

He moved his tongue. I couldn't believe what I had just seen. After the initial shock, I ran around the house to tell Jenny and the girls, who were wondering what had just happened. Everyone hugged Luke; I held him and didn't want to let go. From that day forward, I knew he understood, and more importantly, I was certain that he would continue to improve. I was more determined than ever to work with Luke, coach him, motivate him, and do whatever I could to pull more out of him. Together, we were going to shock the world.

I had coached at Texas Tech for 23 years, but my most important coaching was taking place with Luke. Luke continued to have PT, OT, and speech multiple times a week. I spent hours on the phone and visited with experts to find out what we could do next for Luke.

I came across the neurological recovery center in Fort Worth through a friend. Beginning in August of 2017, I drove 4.5 hours to Fort Worth every Wednesday and returned each Friday for therapy at the NRC nearly every week for two years.

The staff was a blessing, and we were able to get Luke on the Lokomat three days a week. The Lokomat is a robotic machine that allows the patient to walk. Luke needed to be upright as much as possible, and the walking motion seemed to agree with him—well, not the first time. Luke and Jenny had traveled to Fort Worth to try out the Lokomat in November of 2016, and within 10 minutes of walking, he moved his legs awkwardly. The therapist immediately stopped the machine and Jenny took Luke back to the hotel. He continued to be agitated, occasionally crying out. Jenny assumed it was another ear infection. The next morning, Jenny took Luke back to the NRC to try out the Lokomat, but the therapist noticed Luke's leg was swollen. An hour later it was revealed that Luke had broken his femur. We were much more observant after that and took steps to make sure he wasn't straining too much on the machine.

We tried a little bit of everything; if I thought walking to New York would help, I would have done it. We spent time in the hyperbaric oxygen chamber, had multiple stem cell infusions and two weeks of laser therapy, and purchased two lasers.

People have asked many times which therapy benefited Luke the most. That question is impossible to answer. I believe that each of them as well as PT, OT, and speech contributed to his improvement. Therapists and nurses who worked with Luke made a difference, not only because of their knowledge and experience, but by their willingness to build a relationship with Luke.

Jenny and I talked to Luke. One of us was with him all the time and I'm convinced that he felt our love. I played music and talked sports with him regularly. Drew Brees was often his inspiration at therapy, as well as Ed Sheeran, his favorite musician. At night I played classical music for Luke, which he enjoyed.

We took Luke to his sisters' volleyball and basketball

games. We went to Texas Tech sporting events, and almost every day we went on a nice long walk. We also traveled to Phoenix to watch our good friend Kliff Kingsbury and the Arizona Cardinals.

We flew to New Orleans eight times in six years to watch our beloved New Orleans Saints; Drew Brees was Luke's hero. In the fall of 2016, we attended a practice where our family met Drew. Drew told Luke one day he would throw him a pass. The next year he did . . . in the end zone to Luke's buddy Cole, who handed it to Luke. Immediately after the pass, Drew promised Luke the game ball of the Saints, who would beat the Bears. The Saint's staff, coaches, and players were so great with Luke. The game ball sits in Luke's room, reminding us of this moment.

I enjoyed flying with Luke despite the difficulties of traveling with a son in a wheelchair. I was with my hero, so it never felt like a struggle.

Luke continued to make progress. I believe it was a result of all the therapies—the most important of which was love. He was loved by everyone who came into contact with him.

Luke used his voice, his tongue, and his eyes to communicate. I could tell how he was mostly based on his eyes. I knew how he was feeling or if he was uncomfortable, and I even saw many smiles.

My son was a fighter like no other. He constantly amazed me. Every day I woke up thinking today was going to be the day that Luke said a word. And I was going to be by his side every step of the way.

August 16

A friend asked me something over the weekend. He knew it was a dumb question, but asked anyway.

"Which time of the year is the hardest?"

I thought and then paused . . . I came up with this:

> Thanksgiving
> Christmas
> Start of baseball season
> Start of football season
> Start of college basketball season
> Spring break
> Summer
> Summer vacations
> Sundays during football season
> Saturdays during college football season.

The words kept coming.

But the absolute worst is right now . . .

The start of another school year.

I don't read Facebook, I just post.

But I would guess there are posts coming out this week that start with:

> "Where has the time gone?"
> "I'm so excited about her new school year!"
> "Senior year, here we come."
> "Looking forward to this season."
> "Time slowdown."

That last one resonates more than ever. I actually want time to speed up to see what Luke will do next.

Nothing more important for all of us than to live in the moment, and not spend time thinking about the past or worrying about the future.

Easier said than done.

Although I'm not following everyone on social media (it's too hard), I wish everyone a safe and successful school year.

Enjoy every moment. Life is short.

Don't take anything for granted.

Be grateful.

Have compassion.

Remind your children that they have the ability to inspire and impact those around them.

Encourage them to treat their fellow students with respect.

Spend quality time with your children.

And three more things:

Put one foot in front of the other

Fight like Luke

Pray for Luke

- Tim

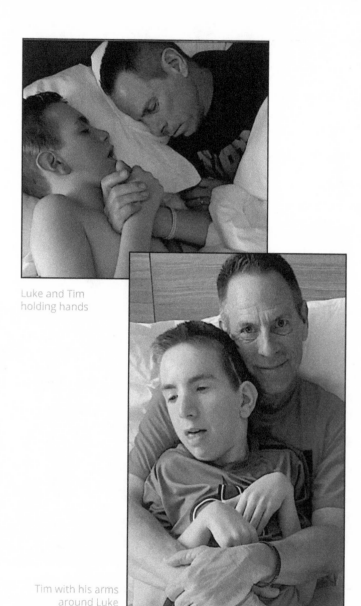

Luke and Tim
holding hands

Tim with his arms
around Luke

02

SUMMER OF 2021

"When a child dies, you bury the child in your heart."
— Korean Proverb[2]

On July 15, Luke and I flew to Portland, Oregon, and then drove with some new friends to Vancouver, Washington to meet the Vancouver Aces, a 9U baseball team. Let me explain how and why we went here.

On December 20, 2020, ESPN aired a story about Luke and me called, "A Father, a Son, and Their Saints." The best storyteller in the business, Tom Rinaldi, chose to finish his career at ESPN by sharing our story. I had reached out to Tom through a friend who also worked for ESPN.

On that day, the New Orleans Saints were hosting the Kansas City Chiefs. Mahomes versus Brees, Luke's two favorite quarterbacks squaring off in the Superdome. Patrick Mahomes was the quarterback at Texas Tech, and every time I walk out on the Texas Tech practice field, I think of one moment: Luke on one knee, captivated by Mahomes's every throw and watching the receiver's acrobatic catches.

One year after Luke's accident, coach Kliff Kingsbury invited Luke and me to watch a practice. This was the first time I stepped on the Texas Tech campus in over a year. Texas Tech was my life before the accident, which made driving on or near the Tech campus impossible for me. Until that day.

Patrick came over to Luke, who had his eyes closed; but I chose to believe that he knew he was in the presence of the Texas Tech football team. Patrick Mahomes has never played a football game for the Kansas City Chiefs without his Team Luke Hope for Minds bracelet on his right wrist. Our family is so appreciative of his unwavering support.

The ESPN story aired in the morning during the *ESPN Gameday* show. I received one special email from Ryan Phillips, who lives in Vancouver, Washington. Ryan watched the story and felt moved to reach out to me. He coaches his son's baseball team and asked if the Aces baseball team could raise money and awareness about brain injuries among children, which we were conveniently equipped to do. Team Luke Hope for Minds is a nonprofit that supports children after brain injuries, the mission and purpose of which I'll share later in the book.

I met the team on a Zoom call and kept in touch with Ryan over the next six months. During that time, the Aces went door to door raising money, putting together a carwash, and shared with their community about a little boy in Lubbock, Texas, and all about our nonprofit.

On July 16, we met the team and their parents for a team dinner, and the next day, we watched as Ryan and the coaches had a hit-a-thon at a beautiful ballpark—their big fundraiser for TLHFM.

At the end of the day, they presented our nonprofit with a check for $31,000. Ryan Phillips, the parent representative, the Aces baseball team, and the Vancouver community will forever be in my heart. I thank God he heard our story that day and decided to pass it forward, honoring Luke and so many others like him.

It was a beautiful trip. Those nine-year-old boys learned a lot about life that weekend, and so did we. An incredible trip . . . and the last one Luke and I would ever take together.

Four weeks later, Jenny and I noticed that Luke wasn't feeling quite right. Our day nurse Cindy took note. She was with Luke up to four days a week since April 2019 and knew everything Luke needed; she became part of the Siegel family. She was an amazing nurse and friend, and even got me into the TV show *Chicago P.D.* and country music. Cindy joined us at Foundation Health and Wellness, where we did the hyperbaric oxygen treatment, as well as other therapies. She joined us for therapy at Trustpoint, an inpatient and outpatient rehabilitation facility. We were together for acupuncture, on walks around the neighborhood, and our many stops for shaved ice at Bahama Buck's.

And now, she was having to give Luke breathing treatments more frequently.

Cindy and I took Luke in for a COVID test because of his labored breathing, but the test came back negative. The next four days Luke looked to be doing OK, but on Saturday, August 14, I insisted he get tested again. Cindy and Jenny took him to the clinic, and when Jenny called, I knew what I was about to hear.

He had COVID.

They sent us home with meds but didn't seem overly concerned, despite one lung showing signs of pneumonia.

The next three days Luke showed no significant signs of COVID. The one thing that seemed strange was that Luke wasn't producing his typical amount of urine. This had only happened twice in the last six years.

I had no idea if this had anything to do with his diagnosis, but I was very concerned.

On Wednesday the 18th, Luke showed real signs of labored breathing, so Cindy and I got Luke in the van and headed to the emergency room.

Ironically, we were assigned to Luke's lucky room #3—but today it didn't feel lucky. Room #3 was all the way at the end of the hall, a foreboding thought. Then, later that afternoon, we were moved to a room on the floor. Part of me wondered why we weren't going to the ICU. Luke's oxygen levels did remain fairly consistent, which certainly kept us optimistic.

Jenny stayed with Luke at the hospital so I could sleep all night for the first time in a week. The past few days I had stayed with Luke and slept maybe an hour or two each night.

I left Jenny and Luke around 7:00 p.m. I drove home in silence as I was too nervous to do anything else. No music. Too tired and too frightened to do anything but drive.

For my entire life, I lived on very little sleep. Growing

up in our house, no one slept in. That even continued in college, and never changed when I coached at Texas Tech, especially during the season.

But tonight, I was so emotionally and physically exhausted, I sat down for a quick bite to eat and then it was right to bed.

But then Jenny called. She told me to get back to the hospital as soon as possible. When I arrived, Luke's oxygen levels had dipped into the 70s, which was extremely dangerous.

A few minutes later they were back into the 90s, but we were aware of his legs moving awkwardly. His legs were kicking out involuntary.

This had never happened before.

I stayed for about an hour and told Jenny I would be back first thing in the morning.

As I began to pull out of the hospital parking lot, I was stopped in my tracks. I had turned the radio on to the Bruce Springsteen channel, and the song that came on the radio was "You're Missing."

I barely moved, and then it took me a few seconds to drive away.

Was this a sign? A coincidence?

This had happened to me once before when I turned on Bruce Springsteen's channel. A few weeks after Luke's accident, I went home to pick up some clothes and spend time with our dog, Saint. I had purposely listened to no music since that fateful July 28, 2015. Nineteen days with no music. I didn't want to hear a sad song, a mournful song, a happy song—any song.

On this day, something forced me to put the radio on as I was leaving the driveway. I fought it for what seemed like a minute, but then I turned on the radio and "Countin' on a Miracle" came on. This was not one of Springsteen's most popular songs, but it spoke to me deeply.

Was that a sign? A coincidence? I don't know, but it was what I needed in that moment.

Back in 2021, I arrived home ready for a full night of sleep.

But then I heard a knock on my bedroom door. Was I dreaming? Unfortunately, it was real. One of Jenny's friends had driven to the house at 4:30 in the morning and greeted me with chilling words: "Tim, get to the hospital. Luke is in the ICU."

I looked in my drawer for a Team Luke shirt, but for some reason I picked the shirt that said, "Luke 4:18, The spirit of the Lord is upon me." Did I choose this shirt, or did this shirt choose me?

I live on 120th Street. When I arrived at the light on 98th Street, I heard a voice.

"You're gonna be alright, but Luke's not going to make it."

I fought that voice for the next few minutes until I arrived at the hospital. The first person to greet me when I entered the ICU was the doctor. She looked at me and quietly said, "I'm not sure if your son is going to make it." I nodded. I already knew.

I hugged Jenny and kissed Luke, and went downstairs to wait for Kate, Ellie, and Alex to arrive.

I walked to the park just across the street from the hospital. I had taken the kids there once when they were much younger. I pictured Luke asking me to push him in the swing.

I had walked around this park in October of 2018, praying that Luke would recover from another brain bleed. We had spent a week in the ICU, and fortunately Luke fought through another setback and recovered beautifully. I walked that day with a purpose. I felt like Luke would recover.

Today, I struggled to walk. My legs had no strength. I felt weak, like I had never felt before.

The girls saw me near the park, and I immediately saw the fear in their eyes. They knew I wasn't doing well. My breathing was accelerated, and it took me twice as long to get to the elevator.

Jenny looked at me and pleaded for me to try to slow down and take a deep breath. I couldn't.

Jenny gave me a Valium to help me relax. But this also did nothing. I was scaring everyone around me. A second Valium did not relax me. My breathing was getting faster and faster. I leaned over and began to feel paralyzed.

Alex and her husband Matt were with Luke, as well as Kate, Ellie, and Jenny.

I needed to get to his room, and I fought my paralysis to get near him. I told him I loved him, I kissed him, and had people nearby carry me out of his room. A nurse looked at me and said that Luke barely had a pulse. It was time, she said.

I collapsed to the ground, just outside of Luke's room.

When I heard someone say that Luke was gone, I began punching the floor.

Minutes later, I overheard a doctor tell Jenny that my vitals were not so good, and that I needed to go to the ER.

Most of the next hour was a blur. I spent most of the afternoon in a hospital bed, but eventually was allowed to go home. Still in shock, I was driven home by a friend . . . without Luke. Our family, our lives, were permanently changed.

August 22

I'm not sure where to begin.

On Wednesday night Jenny called me to come back to the hospital. Luke was struggling to breathe. A very strange feeling came over me as I drove to the hospital. I felt God telling me that I would be OK when Luke was gone. I fought those feelings until I saw Luke. I was worried.

I went to bed at 12 and was awakened by one of Jenny's friends. She told me to get to the hospital as soon as I could. I picked out the shirt that said Luke 4:18. It said, "the spirit of the Lord is on me." I knew. Like was in the ICU when I arrived. There wasn't much time left.

Suddenly I began to struggle to breathe. My hands went numb, my face was tingling, and I couldn't feel my feet. This happened six years earlier on July 28, 2015. But this time it was worse. My blood pressure was high after two Valium. At 8:39 a.m. when I heard the words, "he's gone," I laid face first on the ground gasping for air. The very thing Luke had done the previous hour. I ended up in the ER. I cannot believe. I don't want to believe it. I am in so much pain. Excruciating. Valium has kept me from losing my mind altogether. I

---

have my wife, my girls, my grandsons, and some very special friends, and they need me. Luke is gone, but his legacy will never die. I won't allow it. I was a big part of Luke's life for the last six years, spending almost 24 hours a day with him. But now he will be in my heart until I take my last breath. I remember turning on the radio after three weeks with no music, just after Luke's accident. The first song I heard was "Countin' on a Miracle" from Bruce Springsteen. When I left the hospital last Wednesday night, "You're Missing" came on. A Springsteen song about someone dying after 911. God Bless You. Fight like Luke.

- **Tim**

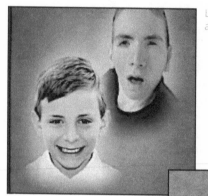

Luke before and
after the accident

Tim's tattoo

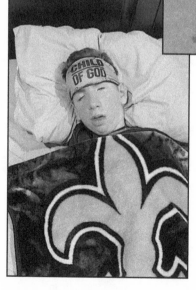

Luke in bed with
Child of God
bandana

03

"RUNNING WITH THE SAINTS"

"I miss you in ways that not even words can understand."
— Gemma Troy[3]

Our family was in shock. A lot of silence, and plenty of tears. My daughter Kate was in the middle of rush week at Texas Tech and actually had a phone interview with a sorority 15 minutes after her brother passed away. Luke took his last breath with Jenny, Alex, Matt, Kate, and Ellie in the room. There were tears, hugs, and more tears. I wasn't involved with the hugs and wasn't with my family because I was rushed to the ER. My biggest regret was that I wasn't there to support our family; I wish I had been able to hold Luke for his last breath.

I suppose I was in shock. It just didn't seem real. I hate the phrase "I can't believe," but for me, I can't believe that my son is gone. He was my shadow until he was nine years old, and for the last six years, I spent almost every waking hour taking care of him.

The first few days were a blur. Jenny slept a lot, and I

cried a lot. I tried my best to be strong for Jenny and the girls.

We received hundreds of texts and calls. Jenny and I are so appreciative of the support we have received in Lubbock, as well as the entire country. So many people who follow our story on Facebook (Pray for Luke Siegel) have offered their prayers and their love.

Three days after Luke passed, I was looking through my email. One of them caught my eye and I ended up reading it multiple times, and each time with tears in my eyes.

Wendy Rae Kerr is from a small town, Idalou, located just a few miles from Lubbock. She is a songwriter, and in her email said that God had encouraged her to write a song for Luke and me.

The song was written as if I was talking to Luke, and the title is "Runnin' with the Saints." The lyrics are beautiful, touching, heartbreaking, and absolutely perfect.

This hadn't been the first time someone offered to write a song for Luke. In 2017, I approached my friend Brandon Gwinn, who I heard sing in church. We met at a coffee shop, and I asked if he would consider writing a song about Luke. I shared with him all about my boy and he took plenty of notes.

He agreed and a month later, "My Boy (Luke's Song)" was born. Brandon wrote the lyrics, the music, and sang the beautiful song.

Luke and I were in Fort Worth for therapy, walking around the beautiful TCU tennis courts when I received the text containing the song from Brandon. I was a little anxious. What if I didn't love it?

I pressed play on my phone and couldn't believe what I was hearing. It's incredible in every way:

My Boy (Luke's song)
(Words and music by Brandon Gwinn)

Your eyes tell the story about the boy you used to be
Running around my memory
You were whole and young and free
You were my boy.

In an instant life forever changed, oh if I had only known
Thoughts of why fill my head and anger makes a home
But you're still my boy.

I'll be here for you.

I've gotta put one foot in front of the other
I won't take no for an answer
I'll be strong and before long
I'll let love kill the fear inside me
Let hope rise and keep on rising
I'll be strong 'cause you're my song.

I found the answers to questions I didn't seek
Never understanding trust is the hardest thing
But you're still my boy
Every day with you is a gift from the Lord
Seeing you fighting through, even tougher than before
Yeah, you're still my boy.

I'll be here for you.

I've gotta put one foot in front of the other
I won't take no for an answer
I'll be strong and before long
I'll let love kill the fear inside me
Let hope rise and keep on rising
I'll be strong 'cause you're my song.

Never lose hope, when you fall don't quit
We serve a God that's bigger than this.

My son, put one foot in front of the other
And don't take no for answer
You're so strong, it won't be long
If you'll let love kill the fear inside of you
Let hope rise and keep on rising
You're so strong, you are my song.

I was so beyond touched at Brandon's love and care he put into the song. This experience only fueled my desire to have music written about Luke and our love for him. So, when I saw Wendy's message and lyrics, I was ready to go.

I got in touch with Wendy that night and told her how wonderful the song was, how blessed we were to have something written about us. I told her I wanted to find a person or a band to write the music and sing it as well. This was my project. I dreamt about Springsteen, U2, or the Lumineers, but I knew that was unrealistic.

This was my priority now. Our song, and I wanted it to

be perfect.

A few weeks later, I was at Luke's gravesite and just thinking about him. Then, a thought suddenly came into my mind.

When we had Andre Agassi at our event in 2018, my friend Bobby brought in from Nashville a husband-and-wife duo called Two Story Road. Andre, who is one of the kindest and most genuine people I have ever met, is so supportive of our mission.

Brandon and Jamie Fraley from Two Story Road were amazing and sang covers from Motown, the '80s and '90s, and their original music. I called Brandon and asked if he would take a look at the lyrics. He was very impressed and said he would get back to me.

A couple of weeks later, he sent me a message, and I was blown away. He wrote the music, and he and Jamie sang "Runnin' with the Saints."

My daughter Kate loves graphic design and putting together videos, so she agreed to make a video to go along with the song, which will become a staple in all of my speaking engagements. The video includes pictures of Luke, our family, and people who inspired Luke.

Runnin' with the Saints
(Words by Wendy Rae Kerr/music by Brandon Fraley)

Runnin' with the Saints now, runnin' with the Saints now.
Yeah, you're runnin' with the Saints now, runnin' with the
Saints now.

I remember the day that Luke was born, couldn't wipe away my smile
A perfect miracle and I thanked God and kissed my little child
Life couldn't get any better than this, how could I ask for more
A lovely wife, three girls, and now a son . . . a picture I adored.

I blinked my eyes and Luke was in third grade having fun at school
We played catch and he'd throw the ball and say "Dad, watch me throw like Drew"
I'd smile and tell him "It's a Brees" as we walked in for the night
He'd kiss his mom and then we'd head upstairs to say our prayers goodnight.

CHORUS

And I prayed each night I'd fall down to my knees
And prayed believing God would hear my plea
I can't believe you're gone
But I'm here holding on to one thing that I know is true
You're runnin' with the Saints now
Runnin' with the Saints now
Cause that's what I prayed for you
I was teaching tennis one day in July like I did most days
Then I got a call but couldn't figure out what they were trying to say
"Luke's been in an accident . . .
we think his nose is broken"
But as I walked into the hospital room

my words were silent and unspoken.

CHORUS

Six years later now we say goodbye 'cause God took you home today
You had it rough but I'm so proud because you fought the fight your way
You'll never know how many lives you've touched and given hope to families
So, until we meet again in heaven
I'll close my eyes and in my dreams, I can see you.

Runnin' with the Saints now, runnin' with the Saints now
Runnin' with the Saints now, runnin' with the Saints now
Yeah I can see you runnin' with the Saints now, runnin' with the Saints now
Have fun runnin' with the Saints, runnin' with the Saints now.

These lyrics are beautiful, but heartbreaking to write down. (To hear this song, go to iTunes). But it was cathartic and so important for me to memorialize Luke in song form, because I would have this forever. "Running with the Saints" was a song about Luke and me and it was the most special gift I had ever received, because we both loved music. This wasn't just music, it was ours, our song.

Through our journey with Luke, I realized writing my experiences down helps me grieve and understand what happened—and not just in music, but in prose.

I remember visiting with a friend when I had just started playing professional tennis, in 1987. I told her that I was thinking about writing about my experiences traveling the world and competing on the biggest stage.

Never happened.

After Luke's accident, I took notes while in the hospital. Notes from Luke's responses to meds he was taking to how I was doing. It became a habit and rekindled my desire to write.

In 2018, I finally made the decision to write a book. I had no idea how it would turn out—if it would even turn out at all. And through perseverance, in the spring of 2019, *It's in God's Hands* came out. It's no masterpiece, but it's a finished product and has been well received. This book was written in the fall of 2018 and chronicles our time in the hospitals, therapies, and our family's journey through the first three years after Luke's accident. And it gives hope to families who have experienced similar tragedies.

One day a couple of years ago, I was driving Luke to Fort Worth to refill his baclofen pump, and to receive more Botox. My love of writing and songs rekindled by the kindness of others and my determination to write a book, I decided to write a song. The idea for the song hit me out of nowhere. I always felt Luke was going to speak. Never a doubt in my mind that he would say his first words in front of me. Every day I thought if he spoke just one or two words, then that would take my pain away. Music in many ways has saved my life over the last seven years, and this was yet another way it could save me.

I jotted down some notes at the gas station, and as soon as we arrived at the hotel, I wrote and wrote and finished the song.

"Take My Pain Away" is a song (or a poem) about the pain I feel every day because of what happened to Luke:

Take My Pain Away

Oh God, please take the pain away
I wonder how long I will have the strength to fight,
To battle every single day
Be strong I'm told, have faith they say
But it's been months, and years so please
Take the pain away.

CHORUS

Oh, Luke I wanna hear you, I wanna know what you're
saying,
What's in your head, what's in your mind
Are you in pain?
But please try not to worry, you have a whole world out there
praying.

I breathe this every moment, every hour
In my belly, in my throat, on my face
Which makes me blue
How and why only makes it worse
But thank you God for friends, wife and girls, and our teams,

for they take the pain away sometimes for a moment or two.

CHORUS

We threw the ball for hours and talked sports for more
You are my hero, the toughest boy I know
What I would give for you to get better, to be more aware
Oh, Luke I will never stop fighting for you
I love you so.

CHORUS

I wake up and wonder is today the day for something new
In your eyes, your tongue, or the sounds I hear
Will it be this week, this month, or this year?
Dear God, all I want is to hear my son speak for that will help
the pain disappear.

Oh, Dear God all I want is to hear Luke speak
For that will take the pain away.

As I write this, I feel my chest tighten because I never had the chance to hear that word I waited so patiently to hear. But I am grateful that we had the chance to "speak" in our way. We definitely communicated with each other, and most of all, Luke knew how much I loved him.

<u>November 7</u>

I talked to Luke a lot today at his gravesite. I told him about the walk we had yesterday in memory of someone who also had a golf cart accident.

And of course, I told him that we were playing our biggest rival, the Atlanta Falcons. My prediction to him was that it would be a down-to-the-wire game because we had a huge win last week and playing your rival the next week would be a challenge.

Then I said something that made me smile. I reminded Luke how upset he got when the Saints lost on a game-ending field goal to Atlanta. The picture of Luke looking out of the back seat window doesn't show the tears in his eyes. He didn't want to talk to Jenny; he was so upset.

Just before leaving Luke's gravesite, my last words to him were, "Hey buddy, let's just hope we don't lose on a game-winning field goal again. You're in my heart."

The Saints lost 27–25 on a last second field goal!

So, I took my dogs on a long walk to help with my frustration. I haven't been to the neighborhood a mile from our house in 12 weeks. Too hard. Reminds me of my walks with Luke in the neighborhood full of kids. We had the same 2.3 mile walk every evening, Luke and the dogs. For some reason I felt today was the day to tackle or walk off my demons. My chest was tight, all the memories hitting me at every corner, and I made sure I walked quicker than normal. But I did it.

Normally, I would need a day to overcome my disappointment after a tough loss by the Saints. I know that sounds silly, but I hate to admit that it's true. Not anymore.

A heartbreaking loss from a football game doesn't compare to a heart that is broken. One foot in front of the other. Taking Luke to Saints games were some of my favorite moments of my life. Today I really have had to Fight Like Luke.

- **Tim**

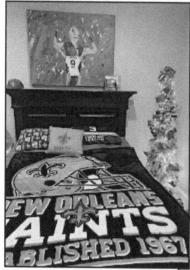

Luke's bedroom

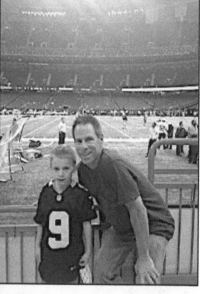

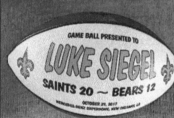

Saint's Game Ball
presented to Luke

Luke and Tim at Saint's stadium

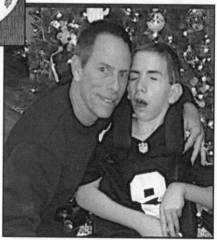

Tim and Luke at Christmastime

04

AUGUST 28, THE FUNERAL

"If people knew how much I truly missed you, they would wonder how I am still breathing."
— Unknown[4]

We scheduled the service for Saturday the 28th, nine days after Luke passed. It was held at the United Supermarkets Arena, home of the Texas Tech basketball teams. I was so relieved that we were able to have it there, because Luke loved being in the arena to watch basketball games, and because there wasn't a church in Lubbock that could accommodate the amount of people who attended.

The night before we held a visitation. My gosh, that night was so emotional. We were blessed to have hundreds pay their respects. Jenny and I hugged a lot, cried a lot, and were humbled to see so many friends.

Earlier that afternoon, I wanted to spend time with Luke. Just Luke and me. I have never been more anxious in my entire life as I was shown which room Luke was in. My heart was racing, my stomach in my throat as I opened the door.

There he was, laying in his casket. So peaceful. Was this real?

His hair was spiked, his hands and face were cold, and he was wearing his #9 Drew Brees jersey. The visitation was very emotional for Jenny. For me, every moment I had a chance to take a breath, my eyes turned to Luke laying in the open casket.

As the last person exited the room, it was Luke, my daughter Ellie, and me. Ellie was holding onto Luke, sobbing. To see your daughter crying because her brother had passed away . . . I don't have the words to adequately describe those heartbreaking moments.

After the visitation, 20 college coaches and friends came to our house to share stories and share their love for Luke.

Our family met in the practice basketball court as the arena began to fill up. The Texas Tech football team, basketball teams, the soccer team, and the tennis team were all there to support. There were also teams from nearby Lubbock Christian University, including the baseball and basketball teams.

Our family entered the arena and sat in the first few rows. Once seated, I stared blindly at the closed casket just in front of me. That moment felt like a terrible dream, but I was painfully awake.

We were blessed to have Pastor Chuck Angel, minister at Turning Point Community Church, and Pastor Ryon Price, minister at Broadway Baptist Church in Fort Worth, Texas. Pastor Chuck has been an inspiration to me for the past year and a half, and Pastor Ryon has been a trusted friend since the day I came to his church in Lubbock just a few months after Luke's accident. They provided us with guidance, support, and love the past few years.

The service began the only way it should: with Luke's hero, Drew Brees, sharing a touching video.

> Luke, I can remember the first time I met you at a Saints practice before a big game, one in which we were probably not supposed to win. And I can remember looking at you and saying, "Luke, you are our good luck charm. Because you are here, I had a great feeling about this one." We ended up winning that game, and there were many more after that, and you had a chance to be a part of the experience and bring us through. You were definitely our good luck charm.
>
> You motivated and inspired us. Your strength, your courage, and your fight motivated us more than you could ever imagine.
>
> To watch the extraordinary love of your family, your father Tim, and your community as they rallied around you was truly awe-inspiring. I know this Luke—I am a better person for having had a chance to know you, and I know the best of you

will live in all of us. God bless you and
God bless your family.

Then my great friend Bobby Banck spoke; he did a
phenomenal job and spoke so eloquently. Bobby shared
that Luke would now become my coach. God would give
me strength and Luke would be my inspiration. Dr. David
Long sang a beautiful rendition of "I Believe in Angels," and
Mandy Buchanan brilliantly preformed Pearl Jam's "Just
Breathe." Both singers sing at Turning Point Community
Church. The message from both pastors was beautiful and
included Luke's incredible impact on so many, the legacy
that will live on forever, and the strength he had throughout
his short life. His life was not about the 15 years he lived but
about the quality of those 15 years.

Then, it was my turn. I walked up to the podium,
glanced at the incredible turnout, and it hit me for the first
time that I wasn't alone, I wasn't experiencing this on my
own. If I were alone, no words would have come out. I had
renewed strength to get the proper words out to honor my
son. As I began, I looked directly at my three daughters. Immediately, I had to look elsewhere because they were unable
to hold back tears. I squared my shoulders and began.

Part of my message was that there are three words that
epitomize who Luke was:

NUMBER 1: FIGHTER

Luke was a sweet, mild mannered little boy. But he was also

determined and loved working hard. He was a fighter most of his life, since July 28, 2015; I cannot imagine a greater fighter in the world.

He overcame over a dozen surgeries, two massive brain bleeds, and a 10-hour surgery for his curved spine. His ribs had been penetrating his pelvis, so two rods and three screws were placed to correct the curvature, which was 75 degrees. He fought every single day from July 25, 2015 until August 19, 2021. Twenty-four hours a day for six years.

He gave everything he had every day in therapy. His strength gave me strength.

NUMBER 2: PLEASER

When Luke was five or six years old, Jenny and I knew that we had a boy who loved to please. Whenever a friend would come over to play with Luke and wanted to play outside, they played outside. If he wanted to play on the X-Box, then that is what they did. Luke loved his friends and especially loved a sleepover.

He was a pleaser with Jenny and me as well. He never wanted to disappoint me in sports, in schoolwork, or anything else. I cannot remember ever getting upset with Luke for making bad choices. Ever!

Well, there is one, but it actually reinforces his desire to please. I was with my tennis team on a road trip. Luke walked into the bathroom in the morning and asked his mom if I was coming home that day. She told him I would be coming home the next day. He left the room, and a few minutes later he came back wearing a Dallas Cowboys jersey. We were huge New Orleans Saints fans, which naturally means we are not fans of the Atlanta Falcons or the Dallas Cowboys. But Jenny and her family have been Cowboys fans forever, and Luke wanted to please Jenny—and made sure it was on a day that I was out of town! He was sweet and considerate like that often.

Luke's last semester of school was in the spring of 2015, the last semester of his third grade. He liked school, but he loved playing football at recess more than anything. One day in May, I drove up to school, parked the car, and watched as the kids played football.

Luke was calling plays, high-fiving players on his team as well as the kids on the other team.

He was having so much fun; I saw firsthand how much he loved playing ball with his buddies. I came home that evening and said to Jenny, "Luke is going to make an impact on a lot of people! You should have seen the way he was leading and interacting with everyone."

About a month after Luke's accident, Jenny had decided to look through Luke's backpack. She was sobbing uncontrollably as she read questions that each student had to answer.

What did you love most about third grade?
Answer: recess
What will you miss about third grade?
Answer: recess and Mrs. Julian

Luke loved Mrs. Julian. A year after his accident, Mrs. Julian asked to come to the house. When she opened the door, she handed me a letter that Luke had written.

> *"Dear Ms. Hunt, Mrs. Cross, and Mrs. Julian, I am writing to apologize for my behavior, I should have acted better. I should have been quieter. I will act better now the whole year."*
>
> *Sincerely,*
> *Luke Siegel*

What had he done wrong? Her answer shocked me. Mrs. Julian told me that Luke did nothing. He wrote the letter for one reason . . . so that the class wouldn't miss recess.

I can't imagine many nine-year-olds who would have written a letter to the principal and his teacher just so that his class wouldn't miss a chance to go outside to have fun. He truly tried to be the shining light in everyone's lives and prioritized others' feelings.

NUMBER 3: INSPIRATION

Luke continues to inspire children and adults every day. The thousands of messages we have received on the Pray for Luke Facebook page shows just how much influence Luke has had on others. I have not gone one day in Lubbock without someone coming up to me to tell me how much Luke has impacted them.

Once, I was walking the dogs when a man got out of his truck. He told me that my relationship with Luke has changed the relationship he has with his own son. I've been stopped at the grocery store, gas stations, restaurants, and at ball games, and the comment I hear most often is: "Your son has made such an impact on our family."

Recently, I was walking on a track on a beautiful spring day and watched as a father was training his son in the 440. The father told me he was training for a meet in the next month. After the boy ran a lap, I walked over to the exhausted runner and said that whenever he feels fatigued to keep pushing. I handed him the "Fight Like Luke" bracelet and told him about Luke's battle. The father knew exactly who I was talking about because he had followed our story.

I began to walk away, and then turned back toward them to say, "I hope this bracelet will inspire you."

They both nodded in agreement.

He truly is an inspiration to so many. It is in these moments that you realize the impact that Luke made and will continue to make.

At the funeral service, I closed by saying that the most incredible thing Luke did in those six years following his accident was that he was able to impact and inspire thousands . . . without ever saying a word.

April 31

Dear Luke.

It's Tuesday afternoon. Our friends and family have gone home after being with you over the weekend. The chairs are back in their proper places, we still have a lot of food, and some pretty flowers sit on the dining room table. The house is quiet. Jenny is running some errands, and the girls are in school.

Your room looks beautiful and clean. There are new large photos of you and the family. But there is a special one that I will look at every day. It is absolutely perfect. Sandra Cooper and Carla Spahr from Timeless Custom Frames created a picture that speaks to me like no other. Jesus with His hand out toward you. My book in the top right-hand corner. And on the bottom left is the verse from Luke 4:18.

For the last six years I was with you nearly 24 hours a day . . . And I loved every minute. We had a beautiful bond before the accident, and that only intensified after July 28, 2015. We have all visited you the last couple of days. Every day that I'm in Lubbock I will be there to think about you, to talk to you, and remind you how you are so loved. I might even mention how the Saints, Chiefs, and Cardinals are doing—and of course our Red Raiders too!

I still sit in our chair, and I still walk the dogs, but we go a different way now. It's not the same without you; they know someone is missing in your room. And I still listen to music. I haven't played Ed Sheeran or classical music yet, but I will. You know that I listen to Bruce Springsteen, and the one song that I have played over and over on my walks is called "I'll See You in My Dreams." One of the lines says, " . . . for death is not the end, I'll see you in my dreams." And guess what, little buddy? You sure will.

Your mom had a dream about you last night. I will think

about you every minute of every day. I will remind everyone to "Fight Like Luke." I'm going to see the Texas Tech football team to give all of them a Fight Like Luke bracelet. They all came to your service on Saturday. They are planning to have a decal on their helmet in honor of you. Isn't that awesome, buddy? You are the greatest fighter in the world. And the greatest son.

- Tim

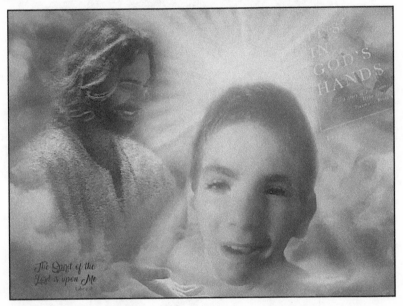

Artwork with Jesus and Luke

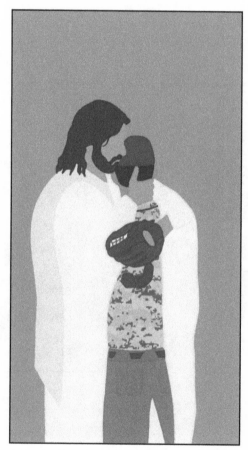

Artwork with Jesus and Luke

05

NOW WHAT AM I SUPPOSED TO DO?

"In the moments of heartbreaking grief, I remember the only reason we have an empty space is because we are blessed with someone who loved us so beautifully it occupied an entire part of our soul."
— Chelsea Ohlemiller[5]

At the end of Luke's service, I paused and said something that was totally unplanned, something I hadn't yet had a chance to think about.

"I've spent the last six years taking Luke to therapy, on Monday there will be no therapy. What am I supposed to do on Monday?"

Monday arrived, and I felt lost. My days had consisted of planning events, talking to parents, arranging speaking engagements, talking to my staff at Team Luke Hope for Minds—but they also included a couple of hours of therapy. Luke being gone had also taken a huge chunk of my schedule away. I didn't know what to do with myself.

Luke's room was originally a two-car garage, which we had turned into a large room with a therapy table, a big closet, and all his equipment. And of course, our chair. Luke and I spent hours and hours sitting in the chair located next to his bed. I held him in my arms during our sleepless nights while we listened to Vivaldi, Ed Sheeran, and Bruce Springsteen, and when I gave him play by play of whatever game was on TV.

That chair was our bond, our safe place, our heaven.

Luke loved sitting with me as much as I loved holding him. I talked to him, and I saw those eyes open wide, and his tongue moving when I asked how he was feeling.

I would often ask Luke to move his tongue if he wanted to hear Uncle Bobby's music. My brother Bobby was a classical pianist, and he played classical music to Luke when he was younger. His tongue always moved for classical music, and for his favorite, Ed Sheeran. It didn't always move for Bruce Springsteen or U2.

That chair was occupied at all hours of the day and night. When Luke's body stiffened, the chair relaxed him. I held him there while giving him his breathing treatments.

The chair is now unoccupied. I have sat in it a few times, but it doesn't feel the same. We had a spiritual relationship in that room, in that chair.

When I stepped foot in that room the next Monday, and I saw his clothes hanging up in the closet, and pictures of Luke everywhere, and his shelf with his New Orleans Saints game ball, and the Drew Brees and Patrick Mahomes signed jerseys . . . I was flooded with emotions. The shock, and then the reality of losing Luke suddenly became overwhelming sadness, mixed with moments of anger. What I didn't expect was real pain in my stomach.

Whenever I would come across a story about a parent losing a child, I wondered how do they survive, how do they move on? Can they ever find joy again?

I am now that parent. And I still don't have the answers to those questions.

I now had two priorities: To do my best to keep Luke's legacy alive by helping other children with brain injuries; and being the best husband and father I could possibly be.

My daughter Alex is 30 years old and has three beautiful sons. Tommy is five and Cal and Miles are three. Alex juggles beautifully between nursing, taking care of three boys, and being a wife to Matt.

Kate is 19, and just finished her freshman year at Texas Tech. She is majoring in public relations, and her dream job is to work for a professional sports franchise, preferably the New Orleans Saints. Kate and I discuss daily the world of Texas Tech athletics, our New Orleans Saints, and her favorite musical groups.

Ellie is 17 and is a senior at Cooper High School. This is her fourth and final year of cheerleading. She is my sweet soul; she loves to talk about her favorite cars and informs me every day about what concert she wants to attend. My girls love music!

Of course, they were all affected greatly by Luke's injury and his passing, which I will describe later in the book.

As I mentioned before, I was with Luke nearly 24 hours

a day for six years. I knew his every move and was aware of what he needed at all times. Jenny even trusted me with his meds, his nutrition, and his overall care. I was his father and his primary care giver. That was what I was, the main thing I felt I was, for a long time.

I recently talked to a former college tennis coach about this feeling. He agreed that coaching became his identity; when he resigned, he felt lost because for so many years, his identity was being a college tennis coach.

I loved coaching. I loved developing my players to become smarter, tougher, and more coachable. My teams played hard and represented Texas Tech University in a very positive way. That was certainly my goal.

But my players knew I was much more than winning tennis matches. Teaching them life lessons, the importance of family, treating people with respect, learning discipline, and hopefully preparing for life after college were among my goals.

I never saw coaching as my identity. It's what I did but wasn't who I was. When I die, my name doesn't need to be on my headstone . . . just the word Father or Dad.

There is nothing I love more than being a dad. But shortly after Luke, I realized not only was Luke gone, but so was my identity. Taking care of Luke had become my identity in ways I never realized. Nothing motivated me more than helping Luke improve.

Regrettably, during those six years my wife and girls saw less of me. The irony is that I left Texas Tech for one main reason: to spend more time with my children. Twenty days after resigning, that all changed.

A thought came to me just weeks after Luke passed. How am I supposed to take care of Jenny and the girls, and somehow take care of me, all at the same time? Jenny was depressed and hurting. I was devastated. And the girls needed their dad to be strong, to make up for lost time.

My story is about grief, love, and family, and helping others through Team Luke Hope for Minds. I had to turn the devastation my family felt at our loss into something that would spread positivity into the world, something that would help others going through similar struggles. Every family deals with something. Grief through a divorce, job loss, or worse—losing a family member.

The journey is best broken up into four parts—three months at a time, ending one year after Luke passed. Each time period brought something different. I experienced different emotions depending on the time of the year, especially during football and baseball seasons. Easter, Luke's birthday, Father's Day, Mother's Day, the anniversary of his accident, the day of his passing, Thanksgiving, and Christmas. I guess you could say . . . all year long. But they all affected me in different ways and brought out the roller coaster of emotions in me each and every day.

AUGUST–OCTOBER 2021

I've read that the more you love, the more you grieve. If that's the case, my grief will be like no other.

I don't entirely agree with that statement because I assume there are parents who loved with all their heart, but found peace, and therefore weren't grieving as hard. Everyone grieves differently—that's a fact. I've seen it in our family and so many families I've shared with.

I haven't found that peace yet. My faith is very strong, so much so that I don't think I could have survived the tragedy without it. But the first few months after Luke passed, I had a hard time focusing on where Luke was, because I was so distraught about where he wasn't.

These first months were incredibly difficult.

Jenny and I were physically in the same house, but we were in our own world. She retreated to her bed, lying there for hours. Working was her only outlet, and she worked only a few days a week at the urgent care clinics. She had a lot of time to think, to cry, and to sleep the day away. Classic case of depression.

Typically, I like to get out and be around people. But what happened to our family was not typical. I fell into a deep, dark hole, and I isolated myself. I thought about Luke morning, noon, and night. In the evenings, I couldn't sleep for more than a few hours, even when taking strong sleeping pills.

My body was used to getting up with Luke in the middle of the night, and I couldn't slow my mind down when I woke up. I didn't want to wake up Jenny, so I spent most every night in Kate's room. Not the perfect recipe for a healthy marriage, I know.

Every night I woke up at three or four and did all I could do to fall back asleep. Eventually, I would look at my phone and read until my eyes grew tired. This went on for the first three months. There was nothing strong enough to keep me asleep and certainly nothing strong enough to take the pain away. I had to adjust to losing the most special time of the day with Luke, the middle of the night, when everyone was asleep but me and my boy! I never felt tired, grumpy, or frustrated. That was our time together.

After Luke passed, those same hours were the absolute worst part of the day. Just me and my thoughts. I tried to focus on my mental health. Therapy, long walks, boxing, visits with my pastor. That helped, but it was all those hours when I wasn't doing therapy or exercising that kept me down.

We have two amazing golden doodles, Jersey and Olive, that are certainly man's best friend. They are with me by the kitchen table, on the couch, on the bed, and most of all, on our walks. On Luke's and my walks, his jogger made him very comfortable and relaxed. I would have Olive on the left of the jogger and Jersey on the right.

The first three months, I struggled to take them on the same walks. They weren't as long, and we definitely had a different path. Those walks were not easy. So many times, I imagined Luke right between them.

By this time, Kate had adjusted well to college. She was a Pi Phi and enjoyed meeting new friends, so she was able to grow into her new environment. Ellie had a more challenging few months; her sister moved into a new apartment the same month that her brother passed away. She spent a lot of time in her room, isolating herself much like I did. I am ashamed to say I was completely aware that the girls needed more of me, but I wasn't there for them emotionally. I was with them physically but that wasn't enough. My girls are strong, resilient, and they know how much I love them.

They are now more likely to express their feelings to me; I am grateful for that.

The one thing we did that seemed to take our minds off everything was to walk the neighborhood on Halloween with Tommy, Cal, and Miles. Our girls loved watching them walk up to the houses asking for candy. I did as well, but my mind drifted to the days I walked with Luke, and I know Luke would have been the best uncle in the world to those boys. Just another adjustment that I had to make to a Luke-free life during those first few months.

October 3

"You're gonna be OK."

On the morning of August 19th on my way to the hospital, I was at a red light not far from our house. At that moment, I heard the words, "You're gonna be OK, but Luke isn't going to make it."

It was so real. So vivid. And also painful to hear. I didn't want to believe it. As I entered the ICU, the doctor came right up to me and said, "I don't know if Luke is going to make it." I nodded; I knew. I heard those words so clearly that fateful morning, and I'm quite certain I know where those words came from. And that does give me comfort knowing that I will get there eventually.

When a friend or stranger approaches, the most common words you hear are, "How are you?" My response for the last eight weeks has been the same: "I'm OK, how are you?"

There is no way my reply is "I'm good." And unfortunately, I'm also far from OK.

I am now in the numb stage. Jenny feels like she is living with a zombie. However, I am doing all I can for myself. Therapy, exercise, sleep, etc. The most difficult part of the day continues to be very early in the morning when my most intense feelings come out. Because I was with Luke all day every day, I am having a hard time filling those precious moments. Our nonprofit takes up much of my time, but I still envision taking Luke to therapy. And walking at the end of the day before watching a sporting event at night.

I am grateful I get to see my three amazing girls almost daily, and those beautiful grandsons of mine.

One of my favorite pictures is this one where I am holding Luke. However, I was doing more than holding him. I was keeping him safe. I was helping him relax. And he was doing the same for me.

Luke,

You are in my heart. And I am doing all I can to put one foot in front of the other . . . I'm trying so hard to Fight Like You. You are my hero. My strength comes from you. You will inspire me forever.

- Tim

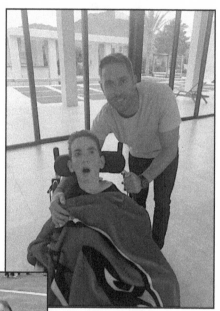

Luke and Kliff Kingsbury

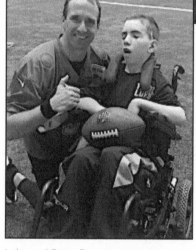

Luke and Drew Brees

06

TEAM LUKE HOPE FOR MINDS

"Don't ask God why He's allowing something to happen. Ask Him what He wants you to learn and do in the midst of it."
— Unknown[6]

After Luke's accident in 2015, I knew that there was no way I could ever coach again. My skills were limited to coaching tennis, and—coaching tennis. That was it. But in 2016, a friend of mine had a suggestion for me: "Why don't you consider starting a foundation?"

My first reaction was that I had neither the time nor energy for something like that. But once I shook off my doubts and started to get the ball rolling, I realized I was wrong. It gave me energy and motivated me, so I made time.

In January 2017, I launched the Team Luke Foundation. I selected board members and had a couple of meetings, but really didn't know how I was going to execute my vision. My strengths are getting in front of people and raising money. Everything else could be defined as weaknesses. I needed someone who could help with the "everything else."

Ronda Johnson was the executive director of Hope-

4Minds out of Austin, Texas. Jenny had told me she had spoken to Ronda on more than one occasion and that she was interested in helping our family. Her friend's son had suffered a non-fatal drowning and she offered to help; she was a friend, a support system. And her continuous efforts eventually turned into Hope4Minds, a nonprofit that could help her friend's son as well as others in Texas. I decided to call Ronda in early June 2017—one of the best decisions of my life!

We spoke on the phone, and the next day I drove to Austin. Initially, I thought she would give me some knowledge on her nonprofit, which I would take back to Lubbock. The funny thing about our meeting was that she said point-blank that her least favorite things to do were . . . getting in front of people and raising money. Maybe that's why she was fantastic at it! She was so brilliant and so capable that I interrupted her and said, "Let's do this together."

She was a one-woman operation. Ronda flew to Lubbock for a meeting with my board, and after only six months, in January 2018, we came together to form the Team Luke Hope for Minds nonprofit organization. I had to keep Luke's name, and Hope4Minds gave the name more clarity.

Our mission is to enrich the lives of children with a brain injury and give hope to their families through support and education; not one penny was given to our family. Ronda's goal with Hope4Minds was to help children in Texas who had suffered a brain injury, and my one request for our joint venture was to help children all over the country.

Ronda would go on to raise money, put on events, and talk to families; almost every day, Ronda is contacted by e-mail or phone by a family needing assistance. Over the first four years we increased our staff to include a Director of Communications (Emily Scorgie), an Executive Assistant (Chelsea Sims), and a Family Service Coordinator (Ruby Sanchez). We have also added new board members and have hired both a consultant and a grant writer to assist us on an as-needed basis. We would not be such a highly successful and helpful company if not for our amazing team.

The scope of this was steady yet staggering. We understood that to help families financially from all over the country, we would have to increase our fundraising—but we could not have predicted how many children needed our support.

In 2021, Team Luke Hope for Minds granted $431,186 to families all over the country. As of June 2022, we have helped families in 36 states. Our organization offers support groups, which include groups for parents and siblings, and brings in respected speakers. It's very important and worthwhile to provide support systems for the entire family, and TLHFM will also pay for counseling for families and help them advocate for their children. We believe that the health and well-being of these children can improve over time if they have access to therapeutic services, adaptive equipment, and educational materials.

In 2021, our average financial assistance request per month was $41,000. During the first six months of 2022, that number grew to $59,000.

We provide financial assistance for:

Therapy

- ADA Home Modifications
- Adaptive Toys
- Durable Medical Equipment
- Auto Adaptive Services
- Medical Claim Advocacy
- Family Counseling
- Family Getaways

Community Resources

- Family Care Packages
- Support Groups
- Brain Injury Resource Guide
- Pediatric Brain Injury Conference
- Educational Presentations

One of our most important events of the year is our annual Pediatric Brain Injury Conference and Resource Fair held in Austin. The purpose of our Making Connections Conference is to connect families and provide resources and education for caregivers. Attendees will explore services and products, as well as listen to presentations on a variety of relevant topics. We offer families travel scholarships to make sure every family who wants to attend can do so.

There is no blueprint for each family when they leave

the hospital. On our journey with Luke, Jenny and I did our own research on different therapies in Lubbock, and we became Luke's number one advocates. We thought we knew what he needed, whether it was nutritional requirements or alternative therapies. But we were always learning and listening to others. I figured out what he enjoyed and what soothed him. And I was never against trying new things.

Luke loved music therapy and pool therapy specifically, but other enjoyable therapies became common during those years. For two years, I drove Luke to Fort Worth every Wednesday and returned home Friday evening. Nearly every week, we travelled over four hours to the Neurological Recovery Center for therapy. The Lokomat was one of the main reasons we made the trip each week, which I mentioned earlier. It is the world's leading robotic rehabilitation device that provides highly repetitive and physiological movement training.

TLHFM partnered with Covenant Hospital to bring the Lokomat to Lubbock. Although our nonprofit supports children 18 and under, the Lokomat is helping patients from all over our region, both young and old. Adults who have a spinal injury, Parkinson's, and multiple sclerosis all benefit from being on the Lokomat. Luke walked with the help of this machine three times a week, and it was obvious to all the therapists how much he enjoyed it.

Therapists were and are the backbone of our operations. I have tremendous admiration and respect for the job they do. Their experience, their knowledge, and their willingness to develop a relationship with their patients is crucial to their development.

They helped me realize that the brain heals. That was the first thing we had to grasp, and once we did, anything was possible. I worked with Luke at home and accompanied him to his therapy sessions. We made it a point not to just sit at home; instead, we travelled, went to dinner, and spent time with friends. He needed this as much as he needed therapy.

Team Luke Hope for Minds has been a blessing to me as much as it has been for the families we've served. Giving hope and resources to a mom or dad, and then to watch them get emotional . . . very powerful and moving.

Much of my time is spent on the phone with parents who recently had their life turned upside down. I've been there, and my presence hopefully offers comfort and guidance. I don't pretend to be a doctor; I simply let the parents know what the experience was like for Luke and me.

Ultimately, I speak to a parent when they are ready. I have visited families in hospitals, at rehab facilities, and in their homes. Even though their pain and anxiety remind me of my traumatic experience, I am truly humbled and honored to be of some assistance.

In my work, I've learned many things about brain injuries. Here are a few troubling facts:

- One in 500 school-age children each year receive a head injury severe enough to be hospitalized.
- Every nine seconds an infant, child, teenager, or adult in the US sustains a traumatic brain injury.
- Fewer than one in 20 people with a traumatic brain

injury will receive the rehabilitation they need.

- Traumatic brain injury (TBI) is the leading cause of disability and death in children and adolescents in the US; the two age groups at greatest risk for TBI are ages 0–4 and 15–19.

We take great care to partner with individuals or companies who desire to be a Mission Partner for TLHFM. Partners play a critical role in supporting the organization, and the generosity of our mission partners allows us to expand the number of families we serve nationwide. In return, mission partners will receive exclusive benefits, access to private events, and more. We invite you to become engaged with Team Luke Hope for Minds, our families, volunteers, and supporters, and to provide hope and help to children who desperately need our services.

I don't ever want to tell a family, "I'm sorry, but we can't help you." Never.

We are excited to announce that as of the fall of 2022, we have started a Team Luke Hope for Minds student organization at Texas Tech University. Ronda Johnson's daughter, Madisen, has helped create this organization and will serve as the president. Tech Team Luke Hope for Minds hopes to bring awareness of our nonprofit and of brain injuries to the Tech campus through education and outreach.

This is not our first experience feeling the generosity of Texas Tech. My good friend Clay Powell is the advisor of the Texas Tech Pike fraternity chapter, and he asked if I would be interested in joining the Pikes. On September 17, 2019,

Luke and I were sworn in as members of Pike. My son is the youngest member of any fraternity ever; he was 13 years old at the time of his induction. As a student athlete at the University of Arkansas, my fraternity was the tennis team. Now I'm a member of the Pike Fraternity!

The Pikes chose Team Luke Hope for Minds as their philanthropy organization. In three years, they have organized a soccer tournament benefitting TLHFM and have volunteered at many of our events, including our 5K fun run and our May event with Demario Davis. It has been an honor to speak at their chapter meetings and a real privilege to see the heart of these young men. We look forward to continuing our relationship for many years to come! It has been wonderful to see the brothers of this fraternity show tremendous passion for wanting to make a difference. Young fraternity members coming together to support a cause because of my son's brain injury is incredibly heartwarming. Team Luke Hope for Minds supports children after brain injuries, but our nonprofit has brought people in our community closer together to help others. That is a very powerful thing, which I am very proud of.

<u>Summer</u>

From the age of seven to 18, summer was my favorite time of the year. I know most kids feel that way because there is no school, and there is the excitement of vacations. But for me, it was the opportunity to play tennis tournaments in Louisiana and the rest of the country. I loved to compete.

When I played professionally, the summer months were my favorite, starting with the French Open, then Wimbledon, and culminating with the US Open. I also loved the summer during my 23 years of coaching tennis at Texas Tech. I was able to take a deep breath following the grueling spring seasons.

AND I got to be with my kids for the majority of the summer.

Summer is different now. It doesn't feel the same, and never will. Luke's accident was on July 28, and he passed away on August 19. July and August are now my least favorite months.

But I plan to make the most of these 61 days, especially for my family, and for our nonprofit.

Today I am visiting two patients in the hospital, and this week we have already received five applications. The families need us, they need me—and I need them as well.

I wish everyone a great rest of your summer.

- Tim

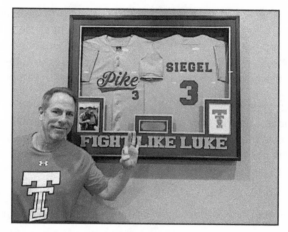

Tim in front of Pike baseball jersey

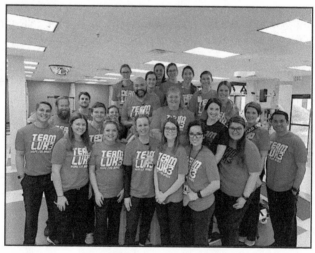

Group of physical therapists wearing TLHFM shirts

07

MY THERAPY

"Grief is like having broken ribs. On the outside you look fine, but with every breath it hurts."
— Unknown[7]

Luke and I had attended many basketball games the past few years, and we would always greet the team in the tunnel on their way to the court.

Just weeks before Luke passed, I watched a few basketball practices with him by my side. I'm convinced that he enjoyed hearing the team, the whistle, and the sound of the bouncing balls, and the players loved having Luke around. Mark Adams, the head coach of the Red Raiders men's basketball team, is a good friend of mine. He has been a tremendous supporter of our mission and was always offering words of encouragement.

He asked me to speak to the team just two weeks after Luke had passed. The entire team and staff had attended Luke's funeral service.

I always felt welcomed to attend practices and games

and to visit with the team in the locker room after their victories. Of course, that was when Luke was with me. Now, it's just me, but the staff and players have welcomed me more than ever. Attending practice became another form of therapy for me. I probably watched the team practice one to two times a week throughout the season, and every time I went, I felt just a little more at peace.

I watched them the way a coach watches practice. The drills, the effort, the energy, what was being said . . . I had my eyes and ears focused on all of it. That hour or two took me away from my pain and into a brighter place each time I was there.

The best part of being at practice was that I was able to spend time with my daughter Kate, who was always smiling at the front desk. She loves her job, loves being around the team, and loves watching practice with me. But what she really, really loves is being at the United Supermarkets Arena, cheering on the Red Raider basketball teams.

The men's games were always packed with the most energetic student section in the country. I loved that Kate wanted me to sit with her at every game; father and daughter cheering on our team was always very special, even though so many of the games brought out mixed emotions for me.

Luke was never far from my thoughts during those moments. As a matter of fact, there were 15,000 screaming fans in our game against Texas, and I remember sitting down while looking at the seat in front of me, when everything went quiet. My focus on Luke seemed to put me inside of a bubble.

Luke and I attended Texas Tech football practices often. This tradition started prior to Luke's accident. I took Luke to watch Patrick Mahomes in 2014, and the memory that stands out is as clear as a blue sky.

Luke and his cousin Easton were sitting side by side watching intently at every throw Patrick made. Luke was in awe and was loving every minute of it. He wasn't looking around or distracted, and he didn't want to leave. He looked back at me every time there was a great catch with his mouth wide open. He was in heaven.

In 2016, Coach Kliff Kingsbury invited us to practice. I walked Luke over in the shade, and one by one every player on the football team patted Luke on the arm or leg. Many of the players told me that they would always pray for Luke.

Prior to the start of the 2019 season, Coach Matt Wells invited me to talk to the team. As I wheeled Luke in front of the team they broke into a "Luuuuuke" chant. Coach Wells was so supportive and cared so much about my boy. That day I asked the team to do me a favor. "Go out this season, and fight like Luke." They loved Luke and I think Luke felt their love.

I ended up attending many practices in the fall of 2021. This was a different type of therapy for me. Being outside and being around the energy of the team was good for my soul.

The night before the second game of the 2021 season, I received a text from Coach Wells. He asked if I would greet the team as they came off the bus before heading into the stadium. I had no intention of going to the game because

I didn't want to hear the cheering and thousands of happy people. This was only four weeks after Luke had passed.

But I was honored and met the team, and as they walked off the bus, one by one, they proudly wore a red shirt with LUK3 on the front. I shook over 100 hands and felt so much emotion as many of the players said some beautiful things to me:

"This game is for Luke."

"Praying for your family."

"We will fight like Luke."

Thank goodness I was wearing sunglasses. My eyes were full of tears.

At the end of the season, Coach Jerry McGuire became the new head football coach. In January 2022, he asked me to speak to his staff. I shared our story and our mission, and why #3 means so much to me. Coach mentioned to me that he has a saying that includes that number. It's called Take 3 University, which means he wants his defense to force 3 turnovers a game.

A few weeks after my talk, Coach told me what he intended to do for the upcoming season.

"The player who proves he is the hardest working, the toughest, and the person who fights like Luke . . . will be awarded #3. He will have earned the right to wear that number." I was speechless when he uttered those words. Such an honor and tribute to my hero.

Texas Tech athletics will always be near and dear to my heart, now more than ever. The Texas Tech basketball teams wore "Fight Like Luke" on the back of their shooting shirts.

The football team had "Luke" on their helmets. The Texas Tech tennis teams wore "Luke" on their sleeves. Texas Tech athletics has named the Luke Siegel Sandlot, located inside the Dan Law Field at Rip Griffin Park, home of Texas Tech Baseball. The McLeod Tennis Center is home to the Texas Tech Tennis Teams, and in April 2022, court #3 was named the Luke Siegel Court.

Ten years ago, Luke threw out the first pitch at the Texas Tech–Texas baseball game (it was a beautiful strike right down the middle). And now . . . I threw out the first pitch at the Texas Tech–Texas baseball game in March to bring awareness to Brain Injury Awareness Month.

The Texas Tech Athletic Department, the coaches, and the teams have been so incredibly supportive, and our family is so blessed and appreciative.

They have provided me with a kind of therapy you can't replicate in an office. The coaches and the players have no idea how appreciative I am to be invited to their practices. Watching the players compete and watching the coaches coach brings me back to my days as the head coach for the Texas Tech tennis team. It also motivates me to continue coaching my new team . . . Team Luke Hope for Minds.

January 8

For the last 20 weeks I have watched sports. Just like I have my entire life. I have watched on TV, and have gone to football and basketball games in person.

But for the most part, I haven't enjoyed one game like I used to . . . until yesterday.

I decided to wear the LUK3 shirt because I had a good feeling. This would be THE good luck shirt.

Even though Texas Tech wouldn't be at full strength, I was convinced with our raucous home crowd, we could beat Kansas. I told myself I was going to bring as much energy to this game as I possibly could. Just like I used to!

What an atmosphere. What. A. Game. What a huge win!

For the first time I allowed myself to really enjoy every moment.

Luke was with me. And with the team. Clarence Naldony played an incredible game. He happens to wear #3. A few months ago, he gave me a signed jersey to put in Luke's room.

After the game I went up to Clarence to congratulate him. He said, "That was for LUKE." Gave me chills.

Thank you, Red Raider Basketball, for lifting my spirits and for fighting like LUKE.

- **Tim**

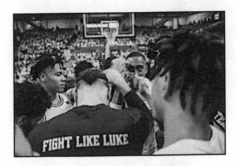
Texas Tech basketball player
wearing Fight Like Luke shirt

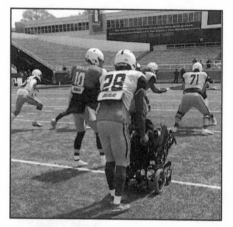

Luke being pushed by Texas
Tech football player

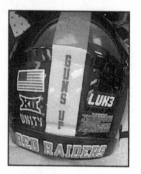

Texas Tech with
Luk3 sticker

08

SPEAKING ENGAGEMENTS

*"Broken things can become blessed things if you let God
do the mending."*
— Unknown[8]

When I was the tennis coach at Texas Tech, I enjoyed getting up in front of an audience to promote Texas Tech and my tennis team. I have always been comfortable speaking, whether it's in front of 10 or 1,000 people, and especially when I am passionate about my subject.

About 13 months after Luke's accident, I was asked to speak at my children's middle school. I was up all night, thinking about my message. It was important to me that my message connect with everyone, from young students all the way up to the elderly.

"Inspirations from Luke" became the focus of my speech. I believe that everyone has been impacted or affected by one of these seven inspirations.

1. FIND YOUR PASSION.

This certainly applies to everyone. We want our children to

eventually find something they are passionate about. Adults who are passionate about their family and their job are great role models for their children.

I lost almost all my passion after July 28, 2015. Nobody was more passionate about family, sports, or Texas Tech than me; somehow, I had to regain what I had lost.

Though people suggested different avenues of passion-finding, I struggled with it. I had to dig deep to regain my passion in a different way. I became passionate about helping my son improve. I also found my passion in helping others. And that passion will never die.

2. DON'T EVER QUIT.

This applies to everyone, every day. There were moments during those years of taking care of Luke when I wondered if I could sustain the pace he needed. When I slept next to Luke, I woke up at least one time a night to turn him. Many nights I just stared at him, hearing every sound and every breath that seemed compromised.

But I never quit, because my little hero never quit.

It is remarkable what your brain can do when your mind is focused on one thing or one person. I lived on very little sleep for six years, but it never bothered me. I rarely missed one of Luke's therapy sessions because I wanted to be there to "coach" him up. My patience never wavered, and my strength remained intact.

Luke's strength gave me strength.

3. LEAN ON FAMILY, FRIENDS, COACHES, TEACHERS, AND COUNSELORS.

For weeks after Luke's accident, I leaned on no one. I didn't answer my phone or the doorbell. Weeks turned into months, and I isolated myself even more. It was destructive and harmful.

Even though I am blessed to have many friends, I felt alone. When I received a text from a friend that said, "praying for Luke," or "thinking of your family today," they gave me comfort. They made me feel like I wasn't on my own in this.

The bottom line is that keeping things inside doesn't help. Find someone you trust and respect and share your feelings. I did that, especially these months following Luke's passing.

And if you see someone who seems withdrawn or depressed, reach out with a text or call. Trust me—these little gestures go a long way toward recovery.

4. MAKE GOOD CHOICES. BE CAREFUL.

Every parent has told their children to make good choices. I remind my teenage daughters to be careful and to make good choices every day.

Unfortunately, I didn't tell that to my nine-year-old son regarding golf carts. I never dreamed that Luke would be allowed to be on a golf cart unsupervised. But it happened, and I will live with that every day for the rest of my life. Every parent should remind their child to make good choices. Kids feel invincible. In one moment, their invincibility is shattered. Emphasize the importance of being careful and making good decisions at all times.

5. HAVE FAITH.

My faith has been tested every day since July 28, 2015.

Speaking in front of people would be impossible. My faith has given me the strength and the comfort to continue to move forward. Prayer has been a staple in my life since that fateful day. Every opportunity I had to speak, or to share our story to an individual, or when I visit with a family, I rely on my faith to make an impact. Despite the loss of my son, my faith in God has never been stronger. On my darkest days I relied heavily on my faith.

6. FORGIVE.

The ability to forgive can set you free. I certainly don't feel free all the time but in order to heal, one must learn to forgive. I know this as well as anyone. I am certainly a work in progress. Some days, I feel lighter and more at peace and then something triggers me and brings me right down the wrong path . . . the path of struggling to forgive.

I am aware that this healing process has many layers. But I'm 100 percent certain that forgiving is the first and most important layer in order for me to heal. Not forgiving someone hurts only the person who needs to forgive. I know because it's time for me to let go, and I will!

7. "LET A LOVED ONE'S LEGACY LIVE ON THROUGH YOU."

Unfortunately, I had to add this one after August 19, 2021. I am going to let Luke's legacy live on through me forever. I feel it is my responsibility to share his story of overcoming. His fight and his determination have given me more fight, and I have never been more determined to impact and inspire others.

The Seven Inspirations from Luke are always a part of my talks because I believe at least one of these seven inspirations apply to us every day. Men, women, girls, boys . . . all of us.

One year after Luke's accident, I was driving aimlessly around Lubbock. I was in a dark place. For some reason, my car ended up in the parking lot of a grocery store I had avoided for a year because Luke's accident was a few blocks from that grocery store; I did everything I could to stay off that street. Except for this day!

I made it a point to park far away from every car in that parking lot. My head was down for a while, and suddenly I was startled from a knock on my window. There was a man in front of my car, and he said words to me that I share every time I speak.

"I'm praying for you. One foot in front of the other!"

Powerful. Poignant.

He never told me his name. He just walked away. He gave me renewed confidence that all I needed to do every day was to simply put one foot in front of the other. It's a cliché, yes, but oh, so true. Putting one foot in front of the other may be one of the most important, useful, and positive things you can do each and every day.

I have used that line quite often in my Facebook posts. We all take for granted that we are able to put one foot in front of the other. I was hopeful that one day Luke would be able to, and I imparted that hope to my audiences.

I also mention another story in my talks. A story of a God Thing.

I was standing next to Luke just outside a basketball gym. He was in his wheelchair, and I was waiting for my daughter's basketball game to start.

I noticed this woman was walking right toward us, but her head stayed down. I've never had anyone walk by us without at least acknowledging Luke or me. Sometimes a sympathetic hello, or a conversation to ask about my son. I've even had people stop and pray.

But she passed right by us and did not look up. Then after walking a few feet toward the gym, she stopped and said, "You were chosen for this." And left without saying another word. I immediately felt the need to tell others what just happened to me. I wrote about this experience, and many of the messages to me was that I was chosen for this. I am not a fan of "Everything happens for a reason," but "I was chosen for this" feels right and true. I will never forget that moment.

There have been so many memorable speeches. What made them so memorable was not what I said, but what members of my audience have said to me later.

"Your talk today changed my life."

"I will pray for your son every day for the rest of my life."

"Thank you for making such an impact."

My goal when I speak is to inspire and make an impact, but often it is my audience who has impacted me. When teenage boys come up to you with tears in their eyes and ask for a hug . . . that is when you know you are making a difference. Never take anything for granted. Be grateful for what you have. And always have hope. My message certainly varies based on my audience, but that is the core of my talks.

Helping others had helped me. Inspiring others has inspired me.

I always close my talk with our video from ESPN or the song made especially about Luke, "Runnin' with the Saints." Nothing impacts audiences more than hearing those words and watching that video.

And most importantly, these speaking engagements help our organization raise money to help even more families. But they also help to bring attention to brain injuries among children when audiences have the opportunity to hear about a little boy who gave everything he had, every single day.

March 26

A special day at Abilene Christian University.

Head football coach Keith Patterson invited me to speak to the team following their morning practice. It didn't take long for me to realize that these coaches and players are a special group.

I got to know Coach when he was the defensive coordinator at Texas Tech. A great man. He shared with the team how his TLHFM bracelet inspired him throughout the season. I visited with many players, including a young man who came up to me as I was leaving. He began to get emotional as he told me that a few of his friends had passed away recently. He was struggling, and living away from home made it worse.

Then he paused and said something that I'll never forget.

"Listening to you today made such an impact on me, and it was just what I needed to help me."

I had woken up at 2:30 that morning and couldn't go back to sleep. I was tired, but as soon as I arrived at practice, I felt a second wind. The team's energy gave me energy. And the young man's words affected me deeply.

I'm so grateful that through Luke I am able to make an impact.

- Tim

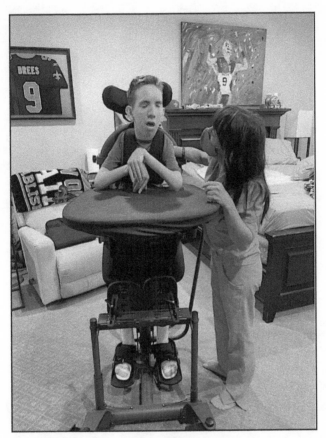

Luke in his room with his therapist

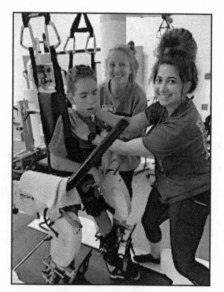

Luke on Lokomat with two therapists

09

NOVEMBER–JANUARY

"The storm that was sent to break you, is going to be the
storm that God uses to make you."
— Unknown[9]

They say firsts are the hardest; my thought is that every holiday, birthday, and anniversary will be the hardest. I don't anticipate any of those days to be lessened as the years go by. I pray that I am wrong.

My favorite holiday has always been Thanksgiving for three reasons: family, football, and food.

But unfortunately, this Thanksgiving felt different—painfully different.

I have three daughters who desperately want to have positive experiences during the holidays moving forward, and it begins on Thanksgiving. They deserve that. So, for them, I focused on having the best day possible.

Our family was blessed to have my parents fly in from New Orleans. They had told me just a month earlier they would not be flying anymore, but I was able to convince them to take one more flight. They needed to see their three grandchildren, and their three great-grandchildren.

Having Jenny, our girls, our grandchildren, and my parents here made Thanksgiving Day slightly better than expected. Everyone enjoyed each other, and the food was delicious.

Football was a good distraction as well. Of course, nothing makes me think of Luke more than when our New Orleans Saints are playing. The Buffalo Bills took it to the Saints, which only heightened my sadness and anger. Certain moments or events trigger my anger now more than ever. I do all I can to suppress those emotions, especially when I'm with the family.

Fourteen years of holding him, playing catch with him, watching football with him, and then pushing him in his chair . . . all of these were gone. I was now left with those memories, and at this time, they were all bittersweet.

The most gut-wrenching moment at Thanksgiving occurred in the early evening when Jenny and I drove my parents to the cemetery. I knew my mom had no intention of getting out of the car. Too painful. The last seven years have drained her physically and emotionally. Every phone call with my mom from the day of Luke's accident to the day he passed resulted in tears.

She would ask how Luke was doing, and whether he was closer to saying a few words, and my answer would always be the same. "He's doing well, mom. Improving every day."

But those exaggerated words didn't make her feel any better. She cried and cried.

I lay in bed at the end of the day remembering our 2015

Thanksgiving, which was spent in Luke's hospital room. I thought about the last five Thanksgivings in which Luke was in his wheelchair, positioned right beside me. I believe he slept through every one of those days.

The day the calendar changed to December, I also changed. My pain intensified, and I felt incapable of snapping out of it. Jenny was depressed, only working and sleeping. I'm now the type of person who likes to communicate feelings and make things better. Jenny, on the other hand, prefers to isolate.

I was reverting to what I was doing before, holding in my emotions. I began to isolate more and more. It was increasingly more difficult to help myself, therefore I felt paralyzed to help Jenny. I was sinking lower and lower, while somehow trying to be the best husband, dad, grandfather, and executive director of a nonprofit. And I was failing miserably.

The weeks leading up to Christmas were much of the same for me. Although these were extremely difficult times, I understood my daughters deserved a good Christmas and a present father.

Kate and Ellie had had very few wonderful holidays since Luke's accident. The attention very often was centered around Luke, and it certainly had an effect on them, but they rarely showed any frustration or impatience. They were sensitive to his needs. But I was sensitive to Kate and Ellie's needs as well, especially during Christmas.

Neither one of them liked the attention that came with a brother with special needs. It impacted them in ways that very few can understand. Quite often during their school activities, Luke was getting all the attention from friends and family. I was there to watch the girls, but he needed to be changed or fed which would keep me distracted from them. And that broke my heart.

Christmas is Jenny's favorite time of the year. She loves to decorate and fills our home with Christmas spirit. She wanted everything to remain the same for this Christmas, which meant Luke's stocking would be hung right next to Ellie's.

All three children have had a small, decorated tree in their room ever since they were little. Luke's tree was decorated in black and gold colors with many different sports ornaments hung, the Saints and Chiefs and Cardinals.

Jenny plans weeks in advance, from the food we will eat to all the gifts for our family and friends. This was her time of the year, and I didn't want to ruin it. We both knew how the other felt, but this December we put our sadness aside, for our girls.

On Christmas Eve the plan was to wrap up the gifts, attend church, and then have our annual Christmas Eve dinner. Jenny wasn't in a good enough mood to attend church so I told the girls I would meet them in the parking lot.

I parked, but didn't want to go in. Families got out of their cars with great big smiles, and the thought of a congregation full of happy people made me less than happy. I was just about to text Kate to tell her I was going home when she pulled up right next to me. It was too late for me to back out now. And thank God Kate showed up when she did. Chuck

Angel and the staff at TPCC led a beautiful service, filled with beauty and love. We were blessed that night.

I remember praying for peace. I simply hadn't found any since Luke passed. Instead of thinking where Luke was, I was obsessed with where he wasn't. My goal was to change this mindset not only for myself, but for my family.

Christmas Day was special for Kate and Ellie. They were genuinely happy and so excited to receive their gifts. Jenny and I were happy for them. They deserved everything they received, which was love, gifts, and smiles. Alex, Matt, and the boys also came over, and it made me happy to see those beautiful boys open their gifts. It reminded me of Luke but didn't dampen my mood; I just sat there and remembered giving Luke gifts.

The last five Christmas mornings we had Luke in his chair as each family member opened their gifts. When it was Luke's turn, Jenny opened his gifts, which were shirts, shorts, and pajamas. Most boys get cool gifts like remote control cars, tickets to an upcoming vacation, or cell phones. Luke got clothes. It pained me to know he couldn't enjoy unwrapping a gift he should've been so excited to open, or to watch the expressions on the faces of his sisters as they were so excited to open their gifts. Luke was happier to give gifts than to receive them.

After everyone left, Jenny took a nap. I slowly walked into Luke's quiet room, surrounded by wrapping paper. I sat in our chair. I felt alone, and sad, and missed Luke more than ever.

One thing I realized, even before Christmas, was that

everything had to start with me. Taking care of me, working on me, and getting help for me . . . this had to happen for me and our family.

I felt jumpstarted, and I decided to turn my mentality around and get myself out of my isolation. My self-help consisted of weekly therapy sessions, a couple of meetings a month with my pastor, and continuing to attend Turning Point Community Church every Sunday. My other therapy was walking. I walked for hours and hours with Luke and the dogs, and even walked alone. It hasn't come back completely, but I have faith that walking will become an effective therapy again as I heal.

Sometimes church had an adverse effect on me because of a few words. When Pastor Chuck would speak about suffering or family, or when he would ask the congregation to turn to the book of Luke, the triggers would appear in full force. My mind drifted and my stomach would tighten. I pictured all those Sundays sitting next to Luke, rubbing his leg, and feeling proud of my fighter. It made me feel alone. But overall, the church provided a haven where I could sit in the back with my thoughts as I listened to Pastor Chuck, and more often than not I found peace for that hour.

I also started boxing in January of 2021 with Terry at Right Cross Boxing. The 30–45-minute workout twice a week has literally saved my life. Throwing punches, getting my heartrate up, and relieving stress was the perfect medicine for me.

That and my anti-depressants!

The beginning of the year usually brings renewed optimism. I didn't make a list of New Year's Resolutions, but this year I just asked God to help me find peace. My faith has been tested since July 28, 2015. However, without my faith, I honestly don't know if I could survive. This month I began to dive more into scripture and other books on heaven. This helped me tremendously because quite often, it was a word, a sentence, or a Bible verse that gave me more clarity.

I recommitted myself to more exercise and prayed for better nights of sleep. For over four months I had failed to sleep a full night. I was so tired of being tired. There was no sleeping pill that could help me sleep a full night. And once I was up, all I could do was think about Luke.

The sadness and depression January brought were a nearly insurmountable challenge, but I was determined to set the groundwork for healing. We would not be torn apart by grief.

December 25

It's 5 a.m. on Christmas morning. I woke up at four and couldn't fall back asleep. This is how it has been every single night for 18 weeks.

I have had very specific dreams about Luke. One replays that beautiful moment where Luke was moving his arms toward his therapists, as if to say, "goodbye." That was 14 weeks ago. Then, I woke up yesterday morning to my second dream . . . Luke was three or four years old, and we were throwing a ball in the house. So real. So haunting. And yet, so spiritual.

I have read and heard from friends about how "hard" the

---

first Christmas will be without Luke. But how could it be any worse than what I have already experienced?

Yesterday at around 3:45 p.m., it was worse. I sat in the Church parking lot with tears in my eyes, a lump in my throat, and my heart racing. I noticed happy families getting out of their cars. Smiles everywhere. I didn't think I could handle their joy and positivity while I was still grieving on the inside.

Just then my daughter Kate pulled up, and we walked into Turning Point Church. We sat in the back, which gave me the perfect view of many more happy families. Again, I was struck with the feeling of not belonging.

But then something happened in the next hour. I smiled. The Christmas Eve service was a wonderful blend of beautiful music, and uplifting words. Until the very end . . . when Pastor Chuck mentioned the word COVID.

Every day, all day, I am subjected to COVID talk. We all are, but not everyone has been affected in the same way. COVID had not taken their son's life.

I slept in Luke's bed last night for only the second time since he passed. Something came over me to come into his room. For the first time, being in his room brought me closer to him.

Today is going to be hard. So hard.

The stocking under the mantle that says LUKE makes my heart hurt, but I'm so grateful for the names next to it. It will be a good day. My beautiful girls deserve it. God knows, Jenny deserves it.

I hope today is a good day for you.

Merry Christmas.

- Tim

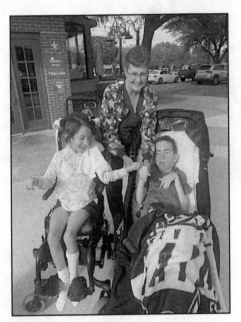

Ava and Luke with nurse

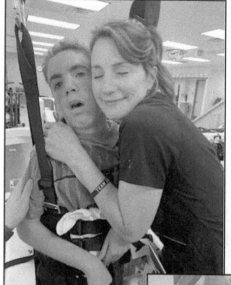

Luke on Lokomat with therapist

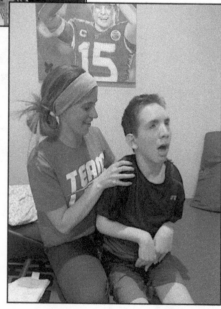

Luke and therapist wearing TLHFM shirt

10

THE GRAVESITE

"Time passes . . . but not one day goes by that you are not here in my heart. The day you died was not just a date on a calendar . . . it was the day when my very existence changed forever."
— Unknown[10]

The first few months I went to the gravesite almost every day. It was my time to sit on the bench and talk to Luke, think about him, and shed a few tears. The first 30 days or so left me in a worse state after leaving than when I arrived. It just didn't seem real. My stomach hurt, and my heart was broken.

Eventually I managed to sit on the bench, stare at all the beautiful flowers, and get back in my car without feeling sick to my stomach. It also helped to know that Luke's legacy would continue.

On more than one occasion, people have come up to me after visiting their loved ones and told me how much Luke meant to them. Once, a mom walked over with tears in her eyes and said, "Your son has impacted my life more than you'll ever know." Occurrences like this made me feel blessed to have a total stranger take the time to tell me how much Luke meant to her. These moments are never taken for granted; I am so appreciative and humbled by their heartfelt words. For just a brief moment after these encounters I thank God that Luke has made such an impact, but then as I sit on the bench all alone, overwhelming sadness sets in.

One afternoon, a gentleman got out of his car and approached me as I was leaving. He was visiting his son. He told me that he had been following our story for years and wanted me to know that he prays for our family.

Then he paused and said, "It will take some time, but it gets easier."

I asked him how long it took for him. "Fifteen years," he said.

For months I came in the morning, in the afternoon, and in the evening before the sun went down. There was no set time. But one day, after just a couple of weeks, I got up from the bench and said, "Luke, you're in my heart," as I put my right hand over my heart. It felt right, and I leave doing the exact same thing ever since.

One day as I was walking to the car, I took it a step further. I decided to do more than just tell Luke that he is in my heart. I set up an appointment with a tattoo artist and asked him to put a cross over my heart with Luke 8:39 going through the cross.

So now when I look in the mirror, or put my right hand on my heart, I'm reminded of what that tattoo means to me. It reminds me the life I lived with Luke. I look at the tattoo multiple times a day and on one hand I feel close to Luke. He is literally in and on my heart. The tattoo gives me strength. On the other hand, it is a constant reminder of what I have lost.

Lately, when I see a family or an individual stand or sit near their loved one, I wait for them to leave. Then I walk over to see how long they have been grieving. I feel their pain. I pray for that family, and so many others.

Someone recently suggested that I visit Luke less frequently, especially if it made me feel worse. Then she said, "And remember he isn't there. He is in heaven."

But for me I feel closer to Luke by being there. The gravesite has become my safe place, the place where I reflect, reminisce, pray, and talk to Luke. I don't ever leave in a worse state of mind, but I do feel more subdued than anything else. It is a place where I feel a true connection to Luke.

In April, eight months after Luke passed, the Resthaven Cemetery installed Luke's marker. It is a beautiful marker with pictures of Luke before the accident and after.

I waited months to finally see the marker, but when I did, I felt worse. His beautiful smile, the picture with Jenny and Luke, and the one of Luke and me . . . it sometimes takes my breath away.

I still make it a point to visit the cemetery about three days a week. I need to, I want to, and that will never change. But my gosh, seeing the name SIEGEL on the headstone, on the bench, and on the marker just doesn't seem real. Looking at pictures of my son who has passed away, one with his smile, the "Who Dat" on his cheeks, the joy in the dugout, well, they bring back good memories. The others are harder to see, Luke and Jenny, me holding Luke. The more I think about it, all of them are difficult for my eyes to see.

Jenny did a beautiful job picking out the colors of the marker, and the pictures that captured who Luke was. She also added a quote at the bottom which epitomizes exactly the kind of sweet, caring person Luke was each and every day: "If someone tells a boring joke and no one laughs at it, you could laugh at it."

That quote is an example of the kind of heart Luke had every day. On Sundays, Luke would ask if we could buy a newspaper from the same man on the corner because he wanted to help him out by buying multiple papers. He was always thinking of his friends too. In third grade, he asked his buddy to join them to play football at recess. His friend wasn't as confident athletically, so instead he just walked around during that time. One day, Luke took him aside and promised he'd teach him how to play. Soon after, this boy and Luke had their special plays and signals and today he is playing high school football. He told me he would never have played football if it wasn't for Luke. My son always inspired people to reach their potential and be great.

December 26

Dear Luke,

I'm with you at your gravesite, but you already know that because I'm with you every minute of every day.

Ellie and I went to church today, and the word I hear almost every Sunday is the word "suffering."

I'm suffering because I can't hold you in my arms, or take you on a walk, or talk football as our teams are playing.

Would you believe that I'm not even watching football right now?

It is a beautiful Sunday as I sit and stare at your name on the headstone, and on the bench. My God, is that really your name? It can't be!

In my time here today, I have witnessed a woman put up a small Christmas tree next to her loved one, a couple hold hands over their loved one, and just a few feet behind me, there is a woman sitting down in front of her loved one. She just walked by and, in a very sweet voice, said three comforting, beautiful words. "God bless you." She was visiting her two brothers and father that day.

She came back to bring me a bottle of water and mentioned you by name. Your story has been in her heart for years. Then she said something else: "It's so peaceful here."

Luke, you continue to inspire and motivate people all over the world.

And guess what, buddy? The men's basketball team warmed up with shirts yesterday, and on the back of those black shirts were the most special, meaningful words of the year . . . Fight Like Luke.

I looked at my phone when I sat down on the bench and it said 12:03, and the time now is 1:03.

#3 is the one thing that everyone remembers about you. And of course, your fight. You are in my heart and on my heart now that I got that tattoo on my heart! I can picture you shocked that your dad has a tattoo.

Mom and your sisters love you so very much.

Your greatest accomplishment.

- Tim

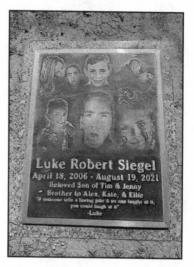

Luke's gravesite

11

FEBRUARY–APRIL

"If you simply cannot understand why someone is grieving so much for so long, then consider yourself fortunate that you do not understand."
— Joanne Cacciatore[11]

Jenny and I spent more time apart during these months than together. We were both working, and then we retreated to separate rooms in the evening. She spent time on her phone, while I wrote for hours. She wanted her space to decompress, and I just needed to deal with sadness alone.

This was not the perfect recipe for a health marriage. But it's how we dealt with our sorrow. I would tell her it was too cold in our bedroom, or that I could only write in Kate's room. They were excuses and I hate excuses. We could have communicated better about what we needed to deal with the trauma. Looking back, we were at the end stages of our unraveling marriage. The stress was too much to handle.

Kate and I were invested in Texas Tech Basketball. We followed both teams as if I were the coach, and she was a player. I really enjoyed talking basketball with Kate. Her background as the point guard on her basketball team made her a real student of the game. She loved to break down every player and every strategy.

Basketball was the perfect diversion for February and March, as was visiting my grandsons. Seeing their smiles and receiving hugs from them was just what I needed.

March is also Brain Injury Awareness Month. My goal is to bring as much awareness to the month of March as I can, and this was not put on hold because Luke was not here anymore. I had a responsibility to the families I serve.

March 3 is known in Lubbock as Team Luke Hope for Minds Day. We encourage our community to wear a Team Luke shirt or the color green, which is the color for Brain Injury Awareness Month. Every day I see Team Luke shirts all over Lubbock, and when I do I feel a strong connection to my community—but also a deep sadness.

Lubbock restaurants have shown their tremendous generosity by giving back to Team Luke Hope for Minds for a day in March. This has become a tradition each of the last five years.

During these months I got back to speaking to parents who needed my support. Each time I received a call from a mom or dad, I was able to put my grieving aside in order to encourage and give hope. That strength came from above, for sure.

On Easter Sunday, April 16, I went to church with Kate and Ellie. Then Jenny, the girls, and I were invited to Jay and Kim Lott's house for a wonderful lunch.

During this time, I was doing OK. The work during the

busy month of March helped me process my grief and also kept me moving. My first Easter without Luke was helped by being with friends and family.

That afternoon, everything changed. I drove to the gravesite to spend time with Luke, and then my mood became somber, mixed with extreme anger. It just hit me suddenly, and it hit me hard. Jenny and I were texting, and my anger about Luke was taken out on Jenny. We texted back and forth and expressed our frustration and anger, and our emotions were sky-high. I felt detached from it all, like it wasn't me who was texting Jenny, but rather a dad who was so full of pain. Unfortunately, however, it *was* me.

I spent the night in a hotel, barely sleeping at all. The next day was April 18: Luke's birthday. He would have been 16. On this day he should have been driving to his friend's house or to a field to throw the ball with me.

I lay in bed most of the day with severe stomach pains. I took a nap. I never take naps, but my heart hurt too much to open my eyes.

The following day marked eight months since Luke's passing. Three days in a row of extreme depression, with the last two days isolated from the world.

I talked to no one on the phone or by text: not Jenny, not my girls, Bobby, or Ronda. These three days were the worst days since August 19.

The month of May couldn't come fast enough, even though grief doesn't just slowly diminish from one month to the next. In fact, eight months later, I felt worse than any of the previous months. Certain days or triggers seemed to take me back to a dark place, one that I can't actually describe. When you're grieving, some days are better than others. Some months bring out more raw emotions. April is certainly that month.

September 15

Luke was moving his hands at therapy. He was smiling and moving them intentionally. I told everyone that he had never done this before.

I was so proud.

Then I woke up. My first dream about Luke since he passed away was last night.

The hardest part of my day is the moment I open my eyes in the morning.

I met yesterday with Pastor Chuck Angel, who spoke so eloquently at Luke's service. He said something to me that I will forever hold onto. He mentioned that my time with Luke, those nights when Luke was wide awake, or those special moments when I could read his eyes and his feelings . . . that the depth of our relationship these last six years was much more than most fathers and sons will ever experience.

A friend sent me this quote that describes it perfectly: "Some days I feel as if I am conquering the world in your honor, and some days I feel as if I'm lost in the heartache of your absence."

Amen.

- Tim

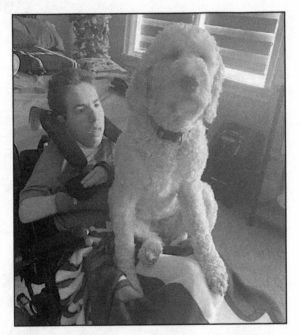

Luke with dog

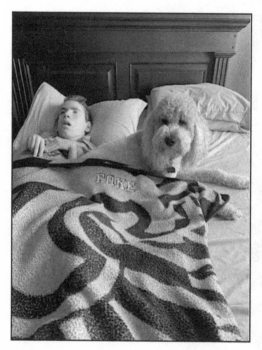

Luke with dog

12

FRIENDS, FAITH

*"Today you could be standing next to someone who is trying
their best not to fall apart . . . So, whatever you do today, do it
with kindness in your heart."*
— Unknown[12]

They say that if you have one true friend who is always
there for you, then you are blessed.

I'm blessed.

Bobby Banck has been a close friend for 46 years. We
met on the opposite sides of the net in the Boys 12 National
Doubles Final. We attended the University of Arkansas together and travelled on the professional tennis tour together.
I was the best man in his wedding, and he would have been
for mine, but he was unable to attend due to his father's
illness.

We have talked on the phone nearly every day for the
past 30 years. Right after Luke's accident, Bobby drove from
Fort Smith, Arkansas, to Lubbock to be there for our family.
He did this multiple times over the first 44 days.

He has been there for me during my darkest of times.

We have a lot in common: our love of sports, our love of our children, and, most of all, our faith. Bobby has reminded me to read scriptures and to trust in God during these painful months. He has a tremendous heart and gives everything he has in everything he does.

I am proud to call him my best friend. We have helped each other and been there for each other, and that will never change.

I am also blessed to have met Jay Lott before Luke's accident. For the last seven years, Jay was always positive regarding Luke's recovery. "Luke will speak one day. It's coming."

He told me that many times.

For the past year, we have met for breakfast almost every week. That hour each week puts me in a better frame of mind, without fail. Jay has challenged me to read scripture that relates to my grief, to consider questions about heaven, and to trust in God. He has been a rock for me during my darkest times and has provided a beacon of hope for so many years.

I met Brett Butler, another close friend, in the beginning of 2021, when we had breakfast in Atlanta. Brett is a former all-star centerfielder. He played for five different teams from 1981 through 1997.

In 1996, Brett was diagnosed with throat cancer. Months later, he had surgery to remove a lymph node the cancer had spread to.

Ten years later, Brett was diagnosed with prostate cancer. He beat cancer three times and later overcame a stroke.

You would think someone who has had cancer three times would be negative and certainly would question his faith.

Just the opposite.

During that first of many breakfasts, I was so excited to meet a baseball player I grew up watching. The Braves, Indians, Giants, Dodgers, Mets—I remember every team he played for. He was fast, tough, and a leader.

Talking baseball with Brett was awesome. But midway through our conversation, he stopped me and said, "Enough about me, your story inspires me. Let's talk about Luke and Team Luke Hope for Minds." I told Brett all about Luke, his love of baseball, his toughness before and after his accident. I shared with him all about our mission and the ways in which we help families all over the country.

Jenny and I flew to Phoenix in October 2021 to watch the Cardinals take on the Green Bay Packers. The highlight of that trip was having lunch with Brett and his beautiful wife, Eveline.

Brett and I have talked on the phone a number of times over the last two years. He has reminded me to surrender to God and to put my trust in the Lord.

In December 2021, Brett came to Lubbock to speak at an event called Hope for the Holidays. He gave one of the most inspiring, motivating, and faith-filled speeches I have ever heard. The audience was in awe of Brett's story and his positive attitude.

Bobby, Jay, and Brett all used the same word . . . trust. They reminded me to put my trust in God and to trust that what I was doing with Team Luke Hope for Minds was God's work. That word trust also applies to me personally. I trust my friends, their opinions, and their advice. I also have trust in me. I know that I have a purpose, and that purpose is to give hope, financial support, and education to families.

I met Simon Robinson in the summer of 1982 in Fayetteville, Arkansas. We became teammates at the University of Arkansas and have been close friends ever since. One of my favorite trips overseas was visiting Simon's family in beautiful Auckland, New Zealand.

I have met very few people who have such a vast knowledge of the Bible. Every time we speak, Simon talks about how Luke inspired him every day, and he never fails to mention where Luke is today.

Simon and his son Kyle, in support of us and our cause, travelled to Washington in July 2021 to be a part of the Aces Fundraiser for Team Luke Hope for Minds. Simon shared some very emotional moments with Luke on this trip, which happened to be our last time travelling.

And then there are friends that came into my life because of Luke. Dave Marcinkowski has been a good friend since his son Sam and Luke played baseball together.

Dave drove me to Fort Worth a few times when Luke was at Cook Children's Hospital, and those conversations were always so meaningful. He was there at my darkest time. In the months after Luke came home from the hospital,

Dave and I talked about Luke, life, and faith at our visits over lunch.

His perspective, words of wisdom, and his friendship helped me immediately during that time, and that help continues today. His relationship with God is always at the core of our conversations, and for that I'll be forever grateful.

A string that connects us all together is our belief in God and our faith in His plan. My faith has always been and always will be a massive part of my life, and in March 2021, I was asked by a good friend if I would be interested in attending a new church. I had no hesitation in finding a new church; in fact, I was looking forward to it. After hearing from my friends, I was confident that this was the place for me. The one thing I knew for certain was that I needed to find a church home that I could attend every Sunday.

Turning Point Community Church is very welcoming, has an incredible group of singers and band members, and is blessed to have Pastor Chuck Angel as its lead minister.

From March through July 2021, Luke and I attended Turning Point almost every Sunday at 10:00 a.m. There was a spot reserved for us in the back.

Luke enjoyed the music, and I was inspired by Pastor Chuck each and every Sunday.

On Luke's 15th birthday, Turning Point showed the ESPN story at all three of their services. The story is on YouTube and is titled, "A Father, a son, and their Saints."

Pastor Chuck had an amazing way of making each person in the congregation feel like he was talking to them. I certainly felt that way.

Pastor Chuck agreed to be one of the two pastors to lead Luke's funeral service. But what he has meant to me personally is hard to put into words. We have gotten together once or twice a month for breakfast the past year, and he has given me comfort, wisdom, and inspiration. Most importantly, he has provided a real friendship.

All of these friends have been there for me spiritually, which is what I have needed these last 12 months.

I am forever grateful.

This Bible verse sums up this chapter beautifully; it's my go-to verse:

> Trust in the Lord with all your heart, and do not lean on your own understanding. In all your ways acknowledge Him and He will make straight your paths (Proverbs 3:5–6).

Putting my trust in Him has not been easy since Luke passed. So much of my focus was on me, my grief and depression, and not enough in trusting God. But this has changed because of the steadfast love and friendship of the people I've mentioned in this chapter. I thank God for Bobby, Simon, Jay, Dave, Brett, and Chuck for constantly reminded me to TRUST and SURRENDER.

April 15

Dear Luke,

I have thought about this day for a few months. Happy Heavenly Birthday, little buddy. You know it's hard for me to put the word happy before the word birthday, but for you I can do it.

Sixteen years old. You should be driving today with your new license and visiting your friends. I know that I shouldn't look back and wonder what if . . . but Luke, it's not easy for me. Tomorrow will be eight months since you passed. The toughest eight months of my life, your mom's life, and your beautiful sisters' lives. My stomach often hurts just thinking about you. I have to choke back tears almost every day.

You were the toughest boy in the world. You taught me so much and gave me strength I didn't know I had. I can only imagine how you would be today. Friends with everyone, well behaved in class, respectful, excited about our future Saints, Chiefs, and Cardinals games, and so much more. You would be throwing the ball with me every day, be the perfect teammate. I would quiz you about the cute girls in your class, and you would get embarrassed. I know you would be the best uncle to your three nephews and you would get along with your three sisters—most of the time. I'm also certain that you would continue to make your mom so proud because of the decisions you'd make.

You were such a beautiful light in this world, BUT GUESS WHAT? Your light has never been brighter. You continue to inspire people every day. Your hero Drew Brees texted me about you! Can you believe the impact you made without ever saying a word? I will continue to remind people to think of you when they see the number three . . . You are in my heart and in my soul every day. I even have a tattoo on my heart to prove it! You are my hero, and a hero to so many. I have told anyone who will listen that there are three words to remember: FIGHT LIKE LUKE.

It was a beautiful thing to watch. Parents and coaches on the field supporting each other. And you should have seen the smiles on those kids when they made contact. Some jogged after a hit, and others were pushed in their wheelchair around the bases. There were regular games on other fields. Young boys playing coach-pitch, and older kids playing kid-pitch. You can imagine all the thoughts that went through my mind. Going back 10 years or more watching my little buddy playing the sport he loved, beaming with pride when he made great defensive plays, and years later participating in the Lubbock Challenger Little League.

Then I thought of something else. Wouldn't it be a great idea if all parents, coaches, and players spent a few minutes before their game and watched The Challenger League? I bet the game that followed would feel and sound different.

I hope everyone has a wonderful Easter weekend. I found these pictures with Luke and the Easter bunny.

I'm at our tennis match after throwing out the first pitch at the TTU baseball game. Our first Easter without Luke. Monday is Luke's birthday. My chest feels tight just thinking about it.

- Tim

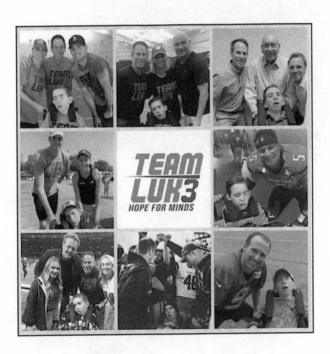

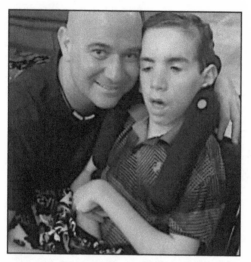

Luke and Andre Agassi

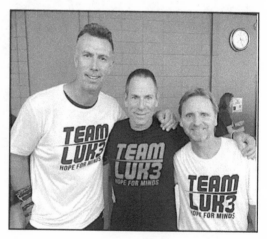

Tim with two friends in TLHFM shirts

13

DEMARIO DAVIS—MAY 11, 2022

"Suffering isn't an obstacle to being used by God. It is an opportunity to be used like never before."
— Levi Lusko[13]

Over the last five years, Team Luke Hope for Minds has hosted a variety of events. These events are one of the ways we raise money to support families whose children have suffered from a brain injury. We are so grateful and blessed to have such talented organizers and so many people who wish to make a positive difference in so many families' lives.

My good friend Bobby Banck has brought some well-known tennis stars to Fort Smith, Arkansas. Andre Agassi, Andy Roddick, John Isner, Danielle Collins, and Brad Gilbert have all been a part of some very special weekends in Fort Smith, and its community has been very supportive of TLHFM.

Ronda Johnson has hosted a very successful golf tournament for years. The tournament hosts over 150 golfers in

Austin each year, which includes an auction and multiple sponsorships.

I have been blessed to have local restaurants donate a portion of their proceeds every year for the month of March.

In 2018, Drew Brees came to Lubbock to speak at the Lubbock Civic Center. Over 1,100 people showed up to hear a wonderful message from Drew. Then one year later, Dick Vitale from ESPN was his usual energetic and enthusiastic self in an event that was held at the United Supermarkets Arena. He gave a wonderful speech and encouraged everyone to support our mission.

In 2021, former All-Star Brett Butler—and my friend—spoke at our event at the English-Newsom winery in Lubbock. He was incredible.

More recently, on May 11, 2022, Demario Davis came to Lubbock for our event at the United Supermarkets Arena. Demario is a three-time All-Pro linebacker and emotional leader for our New Orleans Saints.

Demario became notable on Sunday September 22, 2019, when the New Orleans Saints played the Seattle Seahawks. The National Football League office fined Demario for wearing a headband that was not approved by the NFL. That headband said, "Man of God."

The fine was for $7,017. The city of New Orleans, combined with proceeds from the selling of the headbands, raised a whopping $300,000 for his foundation, Devoted Dreamers, because they loved his message.

His organization equips the next generation of leaders. In 2021, he won the prestigious Bart Starr award, which is given to one NFL player who best exemplifies outstanding character and leadership in the home, on the field, and in the community.

On November 10, 2019, I took Luke to the Saints-Falcons game. The day before that game, we attended the walk-through at the Saints complex. We were fortunate to have been at multiple walk-throughs and this experience every year was every bit as awesome as the game itself.

At the end of the practice, I stopped Demario and told him how much I respected him and mentioned that one day I would love to have him come to Lubbock for an event.

The following day, Luke and I were on the field prior to the kickoff. Luke was asleep in his chair while I was soaking up the atmosphere.

After a while, the Saints had left the field before their player introductions—all but one player. I looked to my right and there was Demario Davis, praying over Luke. A beautiful moment of genuine love.

Just as Demario began heading to the locker room, a gentleman sitting to my left had some great news to share. He told me that he was the photographer for the New Orleans paper, and that he photographed Demario praying over Luke.

It was the most impactful picture I have ever seen. The genuine faith, love, and care that Demario showed over Luke was amazing.

I kept in touch with Demario ever since. He was one of the first people I messaged to tell him that Luke had COVID, and he sent a video to me with an incredibly heartfelt prayer.

In January 2022, I made a very early decision to have Demario come to Lubbock for our event. There was nobody else I would have considered.

Demario arrived in Lubbock from New Orleans on a commercial airline. We had a private plane for him, but it was out of commission just a couple of weeks before the event. All our options were unavailable. I sent him an e-mail explaining our dilemma, to which he replied, "No problem. I'll fly commercial." That right there tells you a lot about Demario Davis.

When he arrived at the airport in Lubbock, I was relieved. In that moment, I knew the event would be a success. We talked football, his faith, and Luke on our way to the hotel.

Demario is a man of faith. He is the leader for the New Orleans Saints, and he is as humble and down-to-earth as any athlete I have ever met.

The event was predictably wonderful; 520 people from the Lubbock community were there to support Team Luke Hope for Minds.

Coach Joey McGuire and Steve Gomez, the women's basketball coach for Lubbock Christian University, spoke very eloquently. Aaron Dawson, whose daughter Joy had suffered a brain injury, spoke about his daughter and the support her family received from Team Luke Hope for Minds.

The highlight of the evening came last. Demario spoke for 17 minutes and every person in the arena was captivated by his every word. His message about Luke was powerful.

He mentioned that God had called him over to pray for Luke before the game against the Falcons. He told Luke that he would be OK, and that he was in God's hands. I was shocked; he had no idea that my first book was called *It's in God's Hands*.

He closed with a message that impacted everyone in the audience.

He told us about Isiah 41:10: "Don't trust anything but me, and I'll take care of you. Nothing can love you the way that God can."

He reminds us that He guides us with Psalm 32:8: "I'll guide you with my eye. As a butler watching for needs. If you don't put your trust in God, He will not guide you. You walk around lost."

And he closed by saying God catches us in Thessalonians 4:17: "We will be caught up together with Him in the clouds."

Demario Davis made this night a resounding success. It was a message we all needed to hear. Friends still come up to me to tell me how moved they were by Demario's speech. One of the best linebackers in the NFL has turned Lubbock Texas into a Demario Davis fan club.

November 17

I was in the lobby as I was approached by one of the employees of Grease Monkey. He noticed the back of my car, which read Team Luke Hope for Minds. He asked if I knew how to get a TLHFM shirt.

"Yes, sir. I'm Luke's dad."

He shook my hand and told me that Luke has been in his prayers for years. I went to the car and handed him my book and a shirt.

When he received my gifts, he paused, looked me in the eyes, and said, "I have lost three children."

Another employee overheard our conversation and said, "Oh my, you are Luke's dad. We pray for you every night." He then told me he lost a child at seven months of age.

The three of us stood by my car, discussing our losses. Three dads in pain. But you would never know it, because these two men were smiling and enjoying their job. I went back into the lobby to pay and noticed a couple waiting by the window. The husband said that he realized who I was and wanted me to know that they also lost a son. Four dads a few feet from each other, all going through the unthinkable. As I drove off, I thought about what I had just experienced.

We never know what the person at a restaurant, a store, at a ball game, or at the mechanic shop is going through. That smile or the kind words from someone could be nothing more than a mask hiding pain. Be kind. Be patient. Smile.

You never know what someone is going through.

- Tim

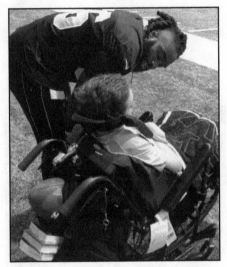

Luke with Saints player

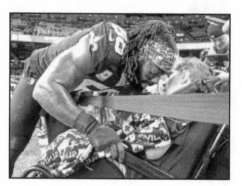

Demario Davis praying over Luke

14

LUKE 4:18, LUKE 8:39

"Grief is like living two lives: one is where you pretend that everything is alright; the other is where your heart screams silently in pain."
— Unknown[14]

I remember sitting next to Luke when he was in the ICU and thinking about the Bible. I then wondered about the Bible verse Luke 4:18. Luke was born on 4-18-06—April 18. We had to go through artificial insemination for Kate and Ellie, so when Jenny told me she was pregnant with Luke, we were shocked. Jenny had a choice when she wanted to be induced, and April 18 became the day that Luke was born. It had to have some kind of significance.

I was driving back with my team from a tournament in College Station when she called me with the good news. Initially I wasn't so sure. We had a two-year-old, a five-month-old, and now she was pregnant! Luke proved to be quite the miracle. We didn't expect him, yet he came into our lives at the precisely right time.

Back in the hospital, I looked at my phone and read Luke 4:18. I was taken back: "The spirit of the Lord is upon me because he has anointed me to spread good news to the poor."

Coincidence?

Luke spread good news to the poor by showing his fight and his determination for six years. He will continue to spread good news through Team Luke Hope for Minds. And I will make sure that continues forever.

The days after Luke passed away, Jenny asked if I knew what time Luke passed. I did not because I was in an awful state at that time. She told me that it was at 8:39 and asked me to read Luke 8:39: "Return home and tell how much God has done for you." Again, I was shocked.

Was this another coincidence?

Every night, I would remind Luke that God was right here with him. Every time I said those words, Luke opened his eyes wider.

Since August 19, 2021, I imagine Luke is with God, talking to him about all the wonderful things he did on Earth. Those two Bible verses have brought us much joy and comfort since his passing.

September 26

I had trouble getting out of bed this morning. Then I received a text from a close friend. He said that my pain is a burden, and that it is a chain wrapped around me. The next line on the text read: "One day those chains will come off, and you will do incredible things."

One day . . . I have to believe that. And I appreciated his heartfelt words.

Today I sat one seat over from where Luke and I always enjoyed our view at church. The seat next to me was open. Minutes later, a woman came up to me and asked if I was waiting for someone. She wanted to make sure that I wasn't saving that spot. In some ways I was waiting for someone, and this hurt me emotionally.

Pastor Chuck's sermon on "Building our Faith" is appropriate for everyone and hits me right in the heart. I do know that without my faith during those difficult six years, I would not have survived. My faith is definitely tested, but I am quite certain that it is needed more now than ever. As I was listening to the sermon and looking around at the congregation, Pastor Chuck put a Bible verse on the screen. That verse was Luke 4:18. I cannot tell you what I felt at that moment. It was hard to hear him say Luke 4:18, but somehow, I felt comfort knowing how often I think of that verse. I had a lump in my throat.

"The spirit of the Lord is upon me and has anointed me to spread good to the poor. He sent me to heal the broken of heart."

Jenny is doing today what she does best: Taking care of patients in the clinic. I'm home alone writing thank you notes, watching football and golf with no volume, and doing my best to remember the words I read and heard today. Luke and I were going to be in Kansas City today for the Chiefs game. He was going to see Patrick Mahomes before kickoff. His tongue would have been moving so fast, and I can picture his smile when #15 walked up to us. Today, instead of having a broken heart, I am focusing on having LUKE IN MY HEART.

- Tim

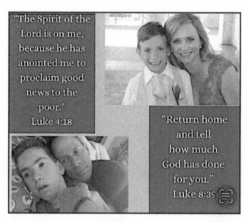

Pictures of Luke, Jenny, and Tim with Bible verses

15

GOD THINGS, PART II

"Grief is the last act of love we have to give to those we loved;
where there is deep grief, there was great love."
— Unknown[15]

In my first book, *It's in God's Hands*, I wrote a chapter called God Things. These were things or moments that happened to me that I believe were not coincidences. I have already shared two God Things that I included in my book that came out in 2019: the man who told me, "I'm praying for you. One foot in front of the other" in the parking lot near the scene of the accident, and the woman who said, "You were chosen for this" at my daughter's league basketball game. Those were two moments that I truly believe were meant to reach us.

There have also been many other God Things that I have shared so far in the book, with more to come in the following chapters.

Once, on December 2, 2021, Ellie and Kate joined me for the Saints versus Cowboys game. I would rather not mention who won that game, but what I do want to talk about is the walk back to the hotel. The three of us were strolling along on the opposite side of the street from the hotel, when I looked up and stared at the sign. We were all silent as we looked at the name of the restaurant, and the number next to the name. Luke333. We couldn't believe what we saw. A restaurant named Luke and the street address was 333: Luke's favorite number, three times! This was a God Thing.

I mentioned earlier that in March 2022, I had the distinct honor of talking to the Abilene Christian Football team after one of their spring practices. Coach Patterson is a first-class man and asked me to share my message to the team and staff in the middle of the field.

After my talk, I visited with a few players and coaches. As I began walking towards the exit, I noticed only one player remaining. He was waiting for me. He told me, "I want you to know I've had a very hard time lately. People close to me have passed away. I just want you to know that your talk today changed my life." This hit me hard.

I have experienced God Things everywhere, from the things I see, the people I meet, special moments, and even text messages.

Andre Agassi is one of the greatest tennis players of all time. He is also one of the most intelligent, well-spoken, and giving men I have ever met. Andre flew to Fort Smith Arkansas in 2018 for our TLHFM event and has continued to support our mission ever since.

One evening a few months ago, I texted him one of

my Facebook posts, and he responded with some incredible words of wisdom.

He knew my pain and heartache and suggested that I watch *The Shack*; just the day before, a friend had suggested the same thing. Then he added, "Our lives haven't crossed for no reason. I am with you."

As I will touch on later, Father's Day has been a sore subject. When I met with a friend over breakfast a few days before, I told him I wasn't sure if I wanted to leave my house, because I didn't want to hear the words, "Happy Father's Day" from anyone.

But deep down, I knew I wanted to hear them from my daughters and if I heard them from anyone else, well, that would be OK too. I ended up going to church and breakfast with Kate and Ellie, regardless.

Later that day, I walked three miles in the West Texas heat before taking Kate and Ellie to dinner. I asked the girls what I could do to be better as a dad, and Kate said something that really impacted me. She said that when I'm with them, I'm not always "with them." I'm physically there, but not emotionally. She was right.

I went to bed around 11:00 p.m. that night, fitful as ever.

Eventually, I woke up, mesmerized by a dream I had. Luke was around seven years old, full of life, with a big smile. We were in the pool and having a great time when I asked him if being in the pool with me was fun. "Yes Dad," he responded, "but I wish Mom was here with us."

Those words have stayed with me ever since. I believe

that Luke was telling me to make sure we were all together. Luke knew the toll his passing had taken on Jenny and me.

I don't think that dream was a coincidence.

The next day, I finally watched *The Shack*, which by then had been recommended by more friends. It spoke to me on so many levels. A father grieves over the loss of his daughter, anger and sadness overwhelm him, and he becomes distant with his family.

He questions many things, including God and heaven. His daughter was a light of his life.

I watched this movie with every conceivable emotion, but by the end tears came streaming down my face.

Then I felt a powerful feeling coming over me. That feeling was that I needed to CHANGE.

The stars had aligned over the last few days. The text I received from Andre, Father's Day with Kate and Ellie, my dream, and finally *The Shack*.

I jotted a few things down while watching the movie and after reading some of the book. These quotes helped me, and I hope they help you:

- "When all you see is your pain, you lose sight of me (God)."
- "Pain is robbing me of joy."
- "I was so lost in my own sadness that I wasn't able to help you with yours."
- "Judging requires that you are superior over the one you judge."
- "When you start to sink, let me receive you."

- "Forgiveness in no way requires that you trust the one you forgive."
- "Don't let the anger and pain and loss you feel prevent you from forgiving him and removing your hands from around his neck."
- "Every time you forgive, the universe changes, every time you reach out and touch a heart or a life, the world changes."

My heart and my eyes were opened, and it led to more healing.

***

Luke was at Cook Children's Hospital in June 2020 for surgery on his spine. He had two rods and 19 screws put into his back to fix the curvature of his spine. We had just moved from the ICU to a room on the floor when a nurse, Emily, approached me with a huge grin.

She told me that she had parked her car in the garage when she noticed that the back of a van had "Team Luke Hope for Minds, supporting kids after brain injury" wrapped on the rear window.

She prayed in that moment to meet Luke because she knew that had to be our van. She became our nurse and helped our family for many years; she was a great addition to our hospital team. We stayed in contact through everything. She reached out to me recently asking if I would be interested in coaching her son for an hour or two on the tennis court, and I look forward to hitting with her son.

***

I was shopping for groceries a few months ago and as I looked toward the checkout, I immediately chose #3.

The woman at the register turned to me and asked if I was Luke's dad. She said that she had hoped to meet me one day to tell me how much Luke and I have impacted her. I went to the car to get her my book and a TLHFM bracelet.

Last week I saw her at the register with the bracelet on her left wrist. She mentioned that she has never taken it off.

***

I had a six-hour drive to Austin last year and stopped at a gas station in a very small town. I got a drink and snack and as I paid at the register, a young woman realized who I was. She wasn't from Lubbock, but she had been following our story on Facebook.

She told me that she prays for us every day and hoped that one day we would meet.

At a gas station in the middle of nowhere!

***

On a particular morning a few weeks ago, I woke up at 2:00 a.m. and I was angry. Some mornings I am sad beyond words. Today, I was angry and tired.

I had planned a week before to have breakfast with a good friend. I considered cancelling because I didn't want to be a downer, but I ended up going anyway because I didn't want to disappoint him.

At breakfast I shared my struggles and started to feel better as we continued our conversation. My friend has tremendous perspective on life and that day he proved that once again. His words hit home: "I think you will continue to struggle until you can forgive. You have to find ways to forgive and when you do, you will truly start to heal."

***

I've had the good fortune to meet many wonderful people in the last seven years who have prayed for Luke and our family. I firmly believe that God places strangers and friends in our lives just when we need them.

Rarely do I go a day in Lubbock without someone coming up to me to say how much Luke has impacted them. When that happens, I am the one who is impacted. I used to believe there are coincidences. Not anymore. They are God Things. I've heard people call them God Winks as well.

February 8

For the last 20 weeks I have watched sports, just like I have my entire life. I have watched them on TV and have gone to football and basketball games in person.

But for the most part, I haven't enjoyed one game like I used to . . . until yesterday.

I decided to wear the LUK3 shirt because I had a good feeling. This would be THE good luck shirt. Even though Texas Tech wouldn't be at full strength, I was convinced that with our raucous home crowd, we could beat Kansas.

I told myself I was going to bring as much energy to this game as I possibly could. Just like I used to!

What an atmosphere. What. A. Game. What a huge win!

For the first time I allowed myself to *really* enjoy every moment.

Luke was with me. And with the team. Clarence Naldony played an incredible game. He happens to wear #3. A few months ago, he gave me a signed jersey to put in Luke's room.

After the game I went up to Clarence to congratulate him. He said, "that was for LUKE." Gave me chills.

Thank you, Red Raider Basketball, for lifting my spirits and for FIGHTING LIKE LUKE.

- Tim

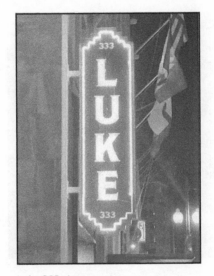

Luke 333 sign

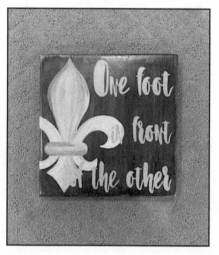

Sign that reads "One foot in front of the other"

16

JENNY AND ME

"We are all just a car crash, a diagnosis, an unexpected phone call, a newfound love, or a broken heart away from becoming a completely different person. How beautifully fragile are we that so many things can take but a moment to alter who we are for forever?"
— Samuel Decker Thompson[16]

Jenny and I were married on July 7, 2001. The first 14 years of marriage were awesome, full of fun, happy times with our wonderful children.

Jenny loved being a nurse and I loved being a coach. But as I've mentioned, I didn't love coaching as much as I loved being a dad. Yes, you can be both successfully, but I wanted more time with the kids. And more time with Jenny.

Jenny and I enjoyed travelling to New York, Las Vegas, and trips with the kids to Florida and New York. One of our few issues was my emotional highs and lows when it came to coaching. My intensity sometimes came home with me. But we had a very good marriage and loved being parents to our children.

Then July 28, 2015 happened.

The first 44 days in Lubbock we were there for each other and so scared we would lose Luke, but the next four months we were apart for most of the time. Jenny was with Luke in Fort Worth the first two months while I visited on Tuesday and Friday through Sunday while doing my best to take care of the girls.

Our roles reversed for a few weeks in October and November. I stayed with Luke and Jenny came home to comfort the girls.

On January 6, five months after the accident, we were all together—physically, that is. Jenny and I were in the same house, but emotionally, we were probably miles apart. I felt we were a great team for our children, but we rarely spent time with just the two of us.

For six years, I felt the need to be with Luke as much as possible. The coach in me had to be there. The dad in me wanted Luke to know I was right by his side.

We juggled our new life as well as we could, but that life was becoming more and more like two close friends just rooming together. We discussed eating out and going on trips together. But in six years, we might have eaten alone together just a handful of times. Those meals produced the same conversations: Luke and what was ahead of us, and what this was doing to our girls.

In those years, we travelled together twice. The first was a disaster because we were both so sad that we couldn't enjoy each other's company. The second trip was slightly better. We had a quick getaway to NYC to see *Hamilton* and Bruce Springsteen on Broadway. But as we walked in Times Square, all I could think about was when we brought Kate, Ellie, and Luke to NYC to see a few Broadway shows.

Both of us were afraid to talk about Luke for fear of upsetting the other. We rarely discussed in depth what we were thinking, which was far different than the first 14 years of marriage, especially for me. Yet at the same time, we were trying to be at Kate and Ellis's school events and there for them emotionally, and for Alex and Matt and their three boys.

Six years of living together, but apart at the same time. I was the communicator in our relationship, but the communication was almost always about our girls and our son, who was never going to be the same.

My days were spent with Luke at home, at therapy, and at ball games. In between those moments, I was driven to raise money and awareness for Team Luke Hope for Minds. Jenny was working part time and maintaining our home and doing both wonderfully.

These days, husbands and wives juggle work and being an Uber driver. Two people passing in the night—but we didn't even do that. Most of my nights were spent lying next to Luke, and even when our nurse was there, I barely slept.

Jenny was concerned that I was wearing myself out with no sleep and questioned whether I needed to be at every therapy. I understood, but I had to be with Luke. I saw it as my ultimate coaching job, and there was no way I was going to give less than 100 percent. I demand 100 percent from my players. I demand 100 percent from myself. And Luke was giving 100 percent.

Jenny and I were doing OK physically, but our son had a brain that was globally damaged. Our hearts were damaged.

Then August 19, 2021 happened.

After the shock wore off, overwhelming sadness, anger, and depression swept over both of us. We truly lost Luke twice. And now we are working on not losing one another.

The year after Luke passed has been hard to describe. But I will try.

My personality has changed. I laugh less, and I was not as likely to be around people.

I tried to throw myself into Team Luke Hope for Minds, which was mostly good for me. On one hand, it was a wonderful feeling to help others, but on the other, I never stopped talking about brain injuries. This took its own kind of toll on my thinking, and often I'd wind up exhausted.

People deal with grief in different ways and at different times. Jenny and I were prime examples of this. But one thing that was the same for both of us . . . was the pain.

And the pain made us feel so alone. I knew that Jenny needed me to hold her, love her, pray with her, and communicate with her. However, I felt so numb that I felt incapable of any of that. And the cracks became crevices we couldn't climb out of.

When you know you should do more for someone you love and you don't, you hate who you are.

Jenny and I both realized that we need to work to regain what we had the first 14 years. And a few months ago, I felt I needed to take more responsibility for making that happen. But we have since come to realize that a lot of broken things cannot be mended.

In any marriage, communication is key. We needed to grieve together and be there for each other—and my gosh, it's only been a year—but we've been struggling through what we mean to each other, and how we have communicated this to the kids. I pray that our pain will lessen in time.

We also know that our girls need us to be strong and positive for them; we lost a son, but they also lost a brother. However, we cannot continue the way we have for so long. So many years of hopes shattered, feelings ignored, and overall grief have transformed this marriage into something that causes more pain than joy.

My wife is an amazing woman and a wonderful mom. Hardworking, smart, caring, and more beautiful than the day we were married 21 years ago. Jenny has just started a full-time job as a nurse practitioner at a new facility, her first full-time job in seven years. This job has been so good for her. It has given her renewed purpose. We all heal in our own ways, and I must allow my wife the liberty of healing through her work, just as I have been attempting to.

We knew that the most important thing we needed to do is lean on God together for our marriage and for our children. We took Ecclesiastes 4:10 to heart for a long time: "If either of them falls down, one can help the other up. But pity anyone who falls and has no one to help them up."

Even though our marriage has transformed into something wholly unknowable, now more than ever, we must lean on each other and rebuild our lives in the most God-serving, purposeful way possible. We are going to lean on God as we both commit to doing our own healing and inner work. If I knew then what I know now... going to counseling, communication, and grieving together would have been a priority.

May 4

I received a call from Resthaven Cemetery that Luke's marker was placed in front of his headstone. I've been waiting for this for eight months. But when I saw it for the first time . . . every emotion came crashing down. Extreme sadness, anger, and everything in between. I looked at his smile, and the picture with Jenny. The one in the dugout, which was the last picture ever taken of Luke, just two weeks before his accident.

A few minutes after I arrived, Jenny pulled up to see the marker. She sat next to me on the bench, crying, and the only words that she was able to get out were, "This is so not fair." No, it isn't. The pain is as severe as it was eight months ago. Sitting next to my wife at the cemetery, looking at our son's marker, it is hard to put into words. There are no words.

- Tim

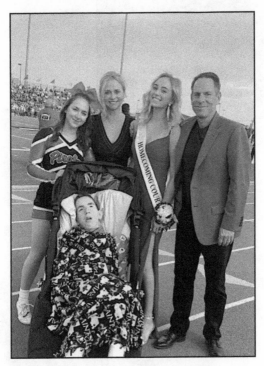

Siegel family at homecoming

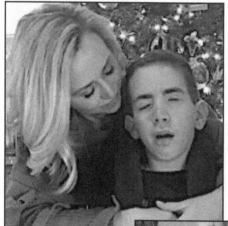

Jenny and Luke

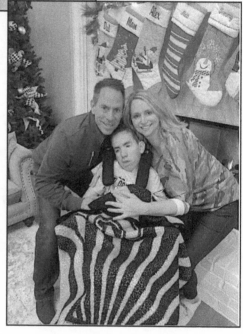

Tim, Jenny, and Luke at Christmastime

17

MY GIRLS

"Children are the hands by which we take hold of heaven."
— Henry Ward Beecher[17]

My daughters are some of my greatest accomplishments and my greatest loves.

My eldest daughter, Alex, is a nurse and a mother of three boys. Tommy is five and Cal and Miles are three. I thoroughly enjoy being a grandfather. They call me "Coach," which I suppose is the perfect name for me. It certainly beats "Grandpa" (for me, at least).

Alex, Matt, and the boys live only a mile from our house, but this year following Luke's passing has made it difficult to visit frequently. The pain at times has been so unbearable that I don't feel capable of being a good "Coach" to my grandsons. Sometimes they make me forget about my pain, but far too often, I find myself wanting to be alone. But I do love seeing them!

I'm so proud of how well Alex has juggled work, marriage, and three energetic young boys. She is also a loving big sister to Kate and Ellie.

Losing her brother, Luke, who she was so very close to, has not been easy for Alex.

As time passes and we heal, I look forward to spending quality time with Alex and her boys as they begin playing sports. Throwing the ball with Tommy reminds me of doing the same with Luke, but I will never let that take away my love of playing catch with them. I long to be the "Coach" they picture me to be.

Kate was an all-state volleyball player but chose not to play in college because she wanted to support the Texas Tech basketball teams. Her passion for basketball started when she was six, and she played AAU ball and was the point guard on her high school team.

Her tenacious passion for Texas Tech Basketball helped her land her dream job at Texas Tech. She is a student assistant and the first person you see when you enter the beautiful Womble practice facility. She loves to talk about the recruits, her favorite players on the team, and the upcoming season.

Kate is majoring in Public Relations and Communications and aspires to work for a professional football or basketball team. I think she has her eyes on the New Orleans Saints! She loves the Saints almost as much as I do. As soon as the schedule comes out, we make our plans to attend at least one game. My favorite story about Kate came in April 2021.

She was so excited to tell me that the Saints had just signed Tyrann Mathieu. And then she said, "Dad, we added a great receiver, an offensive lineman, a cornerback, and now the back end of our defense has improved."

I responded, "Kate, that's the greatest thing you have ever said to me." I was so excited to be able to share this passion with my daughter, because it gave us the opportunity to bond when both of us are less obvious with our affections.

Kate has always been more emotionally reserved. She never liked attention, especially when it came to things like being named the Homecoming Queen. The attention surrounding Luke's accident made her very uncomfortable. She tends to keep her emotions in check.

Following Luke's injury and then his passing, Kate has tremendous empathy for children with special needs. I can see her expression change when she sees someone in a wheelchair. She immediately knows what it is like for the child and the caregiver. This has made her more empathetic and loving to everyone around her.

Ellie is a senior in high school and has been a cheerleader since she was in elementary school. Ellie has such a sweet soul and a kind heart—and a wonderful sense of humor.

In the month that Luke passed, Kate moved into an apartment. The house wasn't the same for any of us, and Ellie really had a hard time adjusting. She spent so much time in her room. Her beautiful smile, which usually lights up a room, was hiding in the dark.

I was aware that Ellie needed her friends now more than ever, and she also needed Jenny and me. Making up for lost time with Ellie was a priority, and so was looking for that smile again.

We spent more time together, visited about school, friends, and life in general. I made it a point to take her lunch to school as much as I could.

Ellie was the middle child in our house for the past 10 years or so. She never complained. In fact, she was always so proud of Kate, looked up to Alex, and loved her little brother with all her heart.

She loves to give hugs, and is the first to say, "Love you, Mom, love you, Dad." We want to offer her the most support we can while honoring Luke's legacy.

My three girls have been through so much. But they are all strong and will always keep Luke close to their hearts. I am incredibly proud of each of them, and I'm certain that they will be there for each other forever. Through it all, we have created a wonderful, dedicated, and supportive family.

October 4

The sun is about to go down as I sit on the bench next to Luke. Sometimes the pretty flowers help my mood, other times it's nothing more than a sad reminder of what lies beneath. Whenever I drive by a gravesite, I'm always aware of those people walking around as they visit the resting places of friends or loved ones. And in that split second, I wonder what kind of pain they were in. Were they visiting someone who lived a long, fruitful life, or a child who suffered a tragic accident?

Here I am tonight, all alone, and I am that person. I read something today that said, "The more you loved, the more you grieve." That explains the levels of my grief.

My good friend Kate was in Arkansas at our event this past weekend. She said something to me that I have felt for the past six years. She mentioned that my relationship with Luke was almost a spiritual relationship. Our beautiful moments in the middle of the night, those hours when I just stared at him, or when I felt such a strong connection . . . it's hard to describe or explain, but it was spiritual.

The sun has disappeared. But I know it will come up tomorrow as I strive to keep Luke's legacy alive. I expected a great deal of emotional pain. I didn't anticipate the physical pain in my chest and stomach. But I know that Luke overcame a different kind of pain each and every day those last six years. I pray that I have the strength to overcome my pain.

- Tim

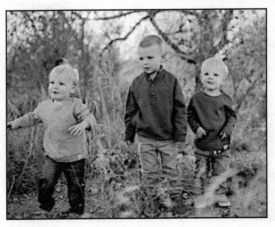

Tim's grandchildren: Cal, Tommy, and Miles

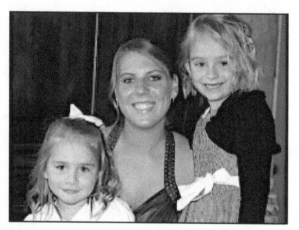

Tim's Daughters: Kate, Alex, and Ellie

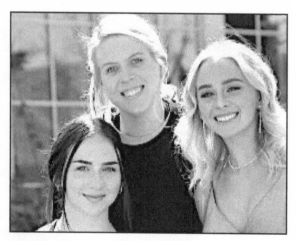

Tim's Daughters: Kate, Alex, and Ellie

18

MAY–JULY

"Some days I feel connected to you as if you are right here with me; then there are days I am overwhelmed by the weight of your absence."
— Unknown[18]

I'm not a big fan of the cold. I would rather sweat in 95 degrees than freeze in 25 degrees. So, when warmer weather arrives, my mood generally improves.

I was extremely busy with two Team Luke Hope for Minds events. On May 7, it was our fourth annual TLHFM 5K Fun Run. We had another fantastic turnout with great music, food trucks, and an appearance from Batman, Catwoman, and the Batmobile.

But this run was different. I didn't get to push Luke with all our friends.

The last time I walked/jogged with Luke was February 28, 2021, when we completed 13.1 miles in the Atlanta Marathon. This was an incredible experience. I had never felt closer to Luke than I did those three hours. Luke and I also did the 5K in Austin two years in a row.

Doing 5Ks and half-marathons was our thing, our bond. I felt his strength giving me strength each and every mile.

May 11 was the event where Demario Davis came and spoke, and one I'll never forget. His speech was one of the best, most spiritual ones I've ever heard. I'm quite sure that there will be more Saints fans in Lubbock than ever before, cheering on #56, the best linebacker in the NFL. Everyone's speeches were motivational and moving and were greatly appreciated by the over 500 people in attendance.

Following the event, Jenny and I spent some time in New Orleans with my parents and brother. My parents, Bob and Gloria, are going strong at 89 years of age. I'm blessed to have wonderful parents, an older brother Bobby, a younger brother Chris, and a sister Victoria.

We do a good job of keeping in touch with each other. Bobby and I love discussing our all-time favorite show, *Seinfeld*, and Chris and I break down college football each year. Victoria has been so supportive and caring during these last seven years.

The last few months were active for our family. The TL-HFM Tennis Tournament took place in Lubbock at the end of May. We were able to raise money and awareness in the tennis community. We then took a quick trip to Austin to see the Eagles in concert.

These events brought me so much purpose and joy, and I often wonder how long I could go without sports or music in my life. They have been such an instrumental form of therapy for me that I cannot imagine my life without throwing the ball around, coaching people, listening to my favorite artists, or otherwise expressing myself in these ways.

I'm determined to keep creating positive memories like this with the people I love the most. I even flew to New York in June to visit friends I haven't seen in 40-plus years and attended Bobby Banck's mom's celebration of life; she was 101 years old when she passed.

While in NYC, my friend Patrick McEnroe invited me to the SiriusXM studio to spend time with one of my all-time favorites, Chris "Mad Dog" Russo. He covers sports on the radio like no one else.

I love music, but sometimes I tune into sports talk radio shows—one of which was his. Years ago, I even had a radio show in Lubbock called *Coachspeak*, which I thoroughly enjoyed. Chris was gracious enough to let me speak on his show about my life and our cause; It was such an honor to speak to a national audience about Luke and our mission. I received texts from friends who heard the show. Christopher "Mad Dog" Russo is an absolute legend on sports talk radio. It was such an honor to share the studio with Patrick, who is a legend as an ESPN commentator, and with Chris.

Meanwhile, Jenny continues to work full-time as a nurse practitioner and is incredibly busy but passionate and good at her job.

We realized that the busier we are, the better, especially when we love what we do.

And God knows I need to stay busy, because every quiet moment . . . my mind goes right to Luke. Nine months have passed, but the pain is just as real, and somehow more intense. Even in the summertime—maybe especially in the summertime—when everyone is out with friends, on vacations, and having fun, it is still a hard reality for me to swallow.

On June 12, I went to the gravesite on a nice warm evening. After spending a few minutes on the bench staring at Luke's marker, I got up to head to the car.

I saw an older gentleman sitting on his chair, and I assumed he was visiting a loved one.

I went up to him and asked how he was doing. He said his wife and grandson passed away just a week apart six months earlier, and that talking to God everyday has helped him cope.

I walked to the car, grabbed my book, *It's in God's Hands*, and handed it to him. He then said something that hit me right in the gut: "It's so hard to let go."

I walked to my car and sat in there for a few minutes. And I realized that what he said is exactly how I felt every day. As I drove off, the gentleman was reading my book. A surreal, sad moment for sure.

So hard to let go.

The next day, I shared this story with a close friend. She sent me this powerful message:

> I can feel your pain. I also see glimpses of
> joy trying to peek out, only to get crushed
> by pain again. To break this cycle, you
> have to want more for yourself. You have

to want to submit your life to God and live
the way He designed you to live. Unfortunately, we only grow through challenges,
trials, and tribulations. He is there with us
to help us through.

I have to want to break it.
I need to break it.
I will eventually break it.
For me. For Jenny. For my girls.
For my boy in heaven.

June 19

I told a friend earlier in the week that I planned to stay at home on Sunday because I didn't want to hear the words "Happy Father's Day."

This quote seems more appropriate for me today:

"Wishing a gentle Father's Day to every father. Whether you are holding onto children, onto memories, or onto hope, we see you."

Gentle instead of *happy*. I like that better.

But instead of lying in bed all day, I am taking Kate and Ellie to church, then to lunch. My girls need a happy father today.

And I need them.

Thirty years ago, I became a dad when Alex was born. Followed by Kate and Ellie, and then Luke.

I chose this picture of Luke sitting in his wheelchair next to me because I had quite a dream last night. I was "happy" because I was pushing Luke in his wheelchair from one store to the next. I loved every moment of being father to him.

Today is 10 months since Luke passed.

To all the fathers, I wish you a Happy Father's Day.

To all the fathers who have lost a child, I wish you a Gentle Day.

- Tim

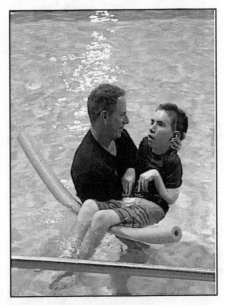

Tim holding Luke in pool

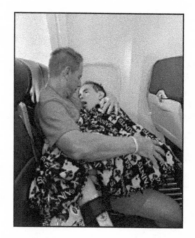

Tim holding Luke on a plane

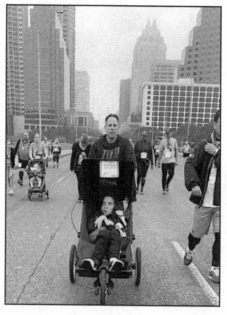

Tim running with Luke at the Austin Marathon

19

SAFETY

"I never knew what strength was, until I saw someone I love battle with a brain injury."
— Anonymous

How protective are you with your kids? With someone else's kids?

This is a sensitive subject because we want our kids to be kids, but our #1 priority should be protecting them from injury. Accidents happen, but so many could have been avoided!

I have a couple rules of thumb:

1. SUPERVISE YOUR CHILD.

Luke was unsupervised on a golf cart while on a city street. Unfortunately, we see so many young children riding golf carts unsupervised. Parents are unaware if their child is safe or reckless. And they are unaware how dangerous golf carts are on a city street.

I have seen children darting out of an alley, nearly hitting a car. And I have witnessed kids running through stop signs with multiple young ones hanging off the back.

When I walked with Luke in our neighborhood, I would very politely remind children to slow down and be extremely careful.

But talking to their parents is actually the better option. Unfortunately, I have heard stories when parents are approached by another parent regarding their child's safety. The response is often, "Thanks, but I'll worry about my child, and you worry about yours."

Shouldn't we be grateful that someone cares? Shouldn't we all look out for the collective safety of our children?

2. TAKE RESPONSIBILITY FOR ALL CHILDREN IN YOUR CARE.

If you as a parent are taking care of someone else's child, that child is your responsibility. What you allow with your own child may not be allowed by another parent.

From 2015 to 2019 we lived in a house that had a pool. The rule we had was that none of our children could swim without a parent present. If they had friends over to swim, they had to get approval from a parent.

This is not an isolated safety precaution that I take. I feel strongly that every child should wear a helmet while on an ATV or golf cart and seat belts as well. It is also incredibly important to wear the helmet correctly, making sure that it is pulled down below the forehead. Just wearing a helmet simply isn't enough; to work properly it must be worn correctly. All safety measures are important to keep our children healthy.

In most states, children must be 16 or have a valid driver's license to drive a golf cart on a city street. But this is rarely enforced.

My attitude about safety did not change after Luke's accident. I was that dad who was protective. But certainly, after his injury, I became more aware and concerned for others.

Friends of mine have asked this question, "What about when we were kids? Did we wear a helmet? We were fearless."

Fair question. But that doesn't mean that we shouldn't teach our children about dangers we may have escaped.

My most important and critical point is simply this: Protect your children from the dangers of golf carts as best you can. Yes, they are kids, but requiring a helmet and demanding that they be supervised is not being over-protective.

I also believe this more than ever: Do what you want with your own children, but when you have someone else's child, you need to be much more cautious. This applies to every possible injury. From swimming, to jumping on a trampoline, to driving, to riding in a golf cart.

Obviously, I am an advocate for golf cart safety. It's my responsibility, my passion, and my calling to bring awareness to golf cart safety. You might be thinking that this could not happen to your child, your athlete, or your neighbor's kid, but it can. In one second.

Researchers from the Center for Injury Research and

Policy at Nationwide Children's Hospital reviewed data from 2007–2017 and found that an estimated 156,100 people received emergency room treatment from golf cart-related injuries. Also, a research team from the Children's Hospital of Philadelphia found more than 63,500 injuries to children in the United States took place between 2010–2019, roughly 6,500 per year. More than half of those injuries happened to children 12 and under.

July is Golf Cart Safety Awareness month in Lubbock. Each year I speak in front of the City Council, and if I can help save one child from a brain injury, then my work will have been worth it.

I will continue to bring up to parents and children the importance of safety. I just recently talked to a parent whose daughter was riding on the back of a golf cart, fell off, and suffered a traumatic injury. These accidents are happening every day. I pray that everyone who reads this will take extra precaution in your car, in the water, and on motorized vehicles.

May 27

I did something a few minutes ago that has kept me frozen in the parking lot.

I went to Covenant ICU to visit a family. This was the first time since the early morning of August 19. As I entered the ICU, my stomach was in knots. I looked down the hall in the exact spot where I was punching the floor when I heard just a few feet away, "He's gone."

I had gone to visit eight-year-old Ethan Perez from Lubbock. Ethan was hit by a truck two weeks prior.

His recovery has been miraculous. He began to speak just a few days ago; I heard him tell his mom that he wants to go home.

Ethan will continue to improve for three reasons:

1. His parents are wonderful. They are by his side encouraging him and loving on him.

2. The staff at Covenant.

3. The support and prayers from our incredible community.

Please keep Ethan in your prayers.

By the way, he is in room #3.

And he is fighting like Luke.

- Tim

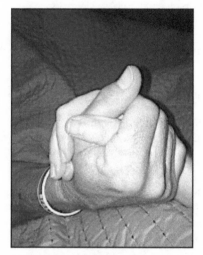

Tim and Luke holding hands

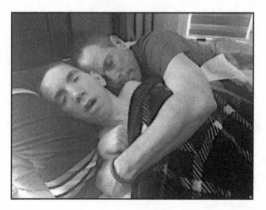

Tim holding Luke

20

GRIEF

"Life is a balance of holding on and letting go."
— Rumi[19]

I have visited with parents who lost a child, and what I've heard consistently is that you don't ever get over it, but you learn to live with it. I'm going to assume this is true, but one year later I'm still learning *how* to live with it. I don't know how long it will take.

I would like to share my story on how I have dealt with my grief—some things that helped, and others that didn't.

Throughout my journey I've read a number of books on grief. I prefer when the author describes his or her tragedy and writes what the experience was like; although the books that point out the different stages of grief are certainly beneficial, they didn't help me as much as I hoped they would, though they did provide a framework for my grief.

These stages apply but not necessarily in this order, because it is well known that everyone grieves differently:

1. Shock
2. Emotion
3. Depressed and lonely
4. Distress
5. Guilt
6. Anger and resentment
7. Resist returning
8. Hope

I read about the three N's of Grief written by Kenneth C. Haugk in his book *A Time to Grieve*:

- Grief is normal
- Grief is natural
- Grief is necessary

Another helpful book was C. S. Lewis' *A Grief Observed*, and Cameron Cole wrote a book called *Therefore I Have Hope: 12 Truths that Comfort, Sustain, and Redeem in Tragedy*. I even had someone send me her book, which is called *Welcome to the Club—I'm Sorry You're Here*. Hope for Grieving Parents, written by Michelle Ruddell. She lost her son over 20 years ago. These books gave me different perspectives on grief. Each book was similar, yet different in its approach in dealing with grief. The overwhelming message is that you need to give yourself grace, be patient, lean on your support system and know that in time you *can* find joy again.

My advice is to google books on grief and read the

reviews. The ones I've mentioned have helped me tremendously, but other types or styles of books may benefit you more.

The difference for me is that I grieved Luke for six years while he was alive. In the first year or two after the accident, I was in disbelief, but at the same time I believed that Luke would improve. I couldn't seem to accept that my son would never play ball again. I couldn't believe that Luke would never walk or talk again.

To be honest, I didn't want to trust what the doctors were telling Jenny and me. My theory was that the MRI didn't measure Luke's toughness or the size of his heart. And it certainly didn't measure my willingness to do whatever I could to improve Luke's quality of life.

The last four years, I saw small improvements, but not significant enough to be certain that Luke was going to walk. But I did hope he'd be able to.

Ultimately, I was OK because Luke knew I would be by his side and we had our special way of communicating. Nothing would ever get in the way of this.

Until Luke was diagnosed with COVID.

Even though we knew how dangerous it was for Luke to get COVID, I had confidence that he would overcome. I don't know if I was naïve or felt that Luke "deserved" to live after all he had endured but on August 19, 2021, at 8:39 a.m., Luke passed away. The only word I have been able to write or say is "passed" when describing what happened.

It just sounds more peaceful.

It has been one year in the life of a father who lost his

only son, the baby of the family. What I have learned this year is that the pain has not diminished, but it does come in waves. Unfortunately, I haven't done a great job in predicting when the really strong waves hit. I'm not sure that is possible, but I am sure of things that have helped.

Initially, I isolated myself from Jenny and my friends. This was necessary for a short time, but I allowed it to last for too long. I had to be around loved ones and friends who "get it." Obviously, if you haven't lost a child, you could never totally "get it," but Jenny and I have tried to surround ourselves with friends who are supportive, loving, and genuine.

There were days I wanted the world, or at least Lubbock, to stop what they were doing and grieve with me, for me. How could everyone just go back to school, sports, and everyday life when I lost my son? Those are the crazy thoughts that have entered my mind, and I assume, others as well.

Here are a few thoughts I've had as I've gone through this grieving process:

1. I CAN'T DO THIS ALONE.

The coach in me needed coaching. Turning Point Church has been a source of comfort, and Pastor Chuck has been a true friend. We all need people surrounding us who support and hold us up when we feel like we can't help ourselves.

I don't know what I would do without Bobby, Simon, and Michael, and, in Lubbock, Dave, Cy, Nathan, Clay, Stan, Jay, and others. I've needed Texas Tech Athletics and my incredible staff and board from Team Luke Hope for Minds.

But most of all, I wouldn't survive without Jenny and the girls.

2. PROFESSIONAL HELP.

I see a therapist once a week and take both an anti-depressant and a sleeping pill almost every night.

For now, I need all three, and I'm not ashamed to admit it. But I will say that getting enough sleep is vital, and my only way of achieving this is with a sleeping pill.

I always encourage people going through life's hard moments to find help. Look for therapists who specialize in trauma and consider what I currently do. I visit with my pastor a couple times per month.

3. EXERCISE.

I box twice a week and walk every day. Boxing helps me release tension and anger and walking is the perfect medicine to gather my thoughts and plan for the next day. Somehow, someway, you need to get out of your bed and do all you can to put one foot in front of the other.

I started with a walk around the block and built up to longer walks. When I walk, I listen to music, which is a must for me. It helps me tremendously.

4. HAVE FAITH.

Although my faith has been severely tested, I would be in a

much worse state without it.

How do people breathe or move forward from tragedy? The answer for me and my journey has been my faith and my trust in God. When I'm at my lowest or struggling to get out of bed, I turn to God. I talk to God; I cry to God.

The bottom line is that losing a loved one is torture. The pain in my stomach has stayed with me for a year. I still can't believe that Luke is gone.

But is he truly gone? I believe he just lives in a different place . . . in my heart.

Find your faith. Find your reason to continue and live for the people in your life. This is how grief can soften and get easier to swallow in time.

October 26

They say grief is like the ocean. It comes in waves. It ebbs and flows. But sometimes it hits you when you don't see it coming.

I was at the checkout line after getting a few groceries. The young boy was bagging those few items when he noticed my Team Luke shirt. He looked at me and said, "Hey, did you hear that Luke Siegel passed away?" That was a wave I didn't see coming.

I woke up this morning at my usual time of around four. Sleeping meds help me fall asleep, but most of the time it doesn't last very long. For nearly 10 weeks, I have dealt with intense feelings every single morning. And for six years, I grieved for my son who was alive.

The waves were there, but I could sense when a big one was

---

coming. Ironically, the first few months this summer, the ocean seemed calm. Luke was responding with his tongue more frequently and much more rapidly. He was enjoying our walks and his therapy on the Lokomat. I wonder if this was the calm before the storm.

I am working hard on me. Therapy, weekly visits with my pastor, medicine, exercise, and occasional lunches with friends. And I'm continuing my mission to help other families, as I have travelled to events three times this month.

And then I realize it's only been 10 weeks.

Jenny and I will be going to Phoenix for a much-needed trip to watch the Arizona Cardinals play on Thursday and spend a couple of nights away from our home. Losing Luke has taken such a toll on both of us in different ways, and at different times. He was our boy. And our life will never be the same.

I have read a couple of books on the stages of grief. I guess you could say there is actually a blueprint for grief. But those authors didn't know the relationship I had with my son these last 15 years. And they certainly didn't know that I basically lost Luke twice. I'm not sure if my grief will parallel with what I've read.

Despite the unpredictable waves of grief, I will make sure that I'm strong enough to not let them overpower me. And on those days that they might, I'll just take that day off.

I was a coach. I'm still a coach. And now maybe, just maybe, Luke is coaching me to be as strong as he always was.

When you see the number 3, take a deep breath, and think of Luke. Hopefully, that will inspire you to fight through your tough times. Fight like Luke. And that goes for me as well.

- **Tim**

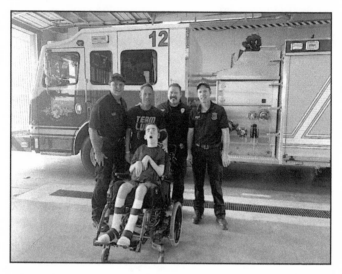

Luke and Tim with firefighters

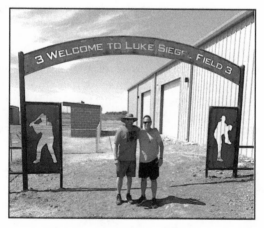

Tim and friend in front of Luke Siegel Field

21

CAN I FIND MY JOY AGAIN?

"Trust in His timing,
Rely on His promises,
Wait for His answers,
Believe in His miracles,
Rejoice in His goodness.
Relax in His presence."
— Unknown[20]

Nearly one year after Luke passed, this is a question not yet answered. There certainly have been moments that have given me reason to smile and even laugh: spending time with Jenny and the girls, playing with my grandsons, cheering for the Texas Tech Red Raiders and my three favorite football teams; the Saints, the Cardinals, and the Chiefs.

But I'm not sure if that was real joy or just momentary happiness.

When Texas Tech Basketball won in thrilling fashion, Kate and I were so excited. But during the game, and especially after, my thoughts went right back to Luke. That is just one of hundreds of examples. I've had so many conversations over the last year about different topics, and while talking and listening, Luke was on my mind.

There is one absolute, and I would like to share it with everyone who is searching to find joy again: You can't achieve joy without help. That help can come from many sources. Lean on a friend or mentor, a pastor, a counselor, a therapist, or books. And don't forget your family.

For me, my close friends have helped me more than they know. The occasional lunch, heartfelt conversations about sports, or deep conversations about Luke have kept me from sinking. I also owe it to Jenny, my three daughters, and my three grandsons to continue to work toward finding joy. They deserve it.

Giving hope and resources to families in need makes me feel alive, which is its own kind of happiness. My life is not a depressing cloud of sadness or grief all the time, and often I find I can enjoy myself.

But am I truly capable of finding joy again? I was that guy who wanted the white picket fence, a couple of dogs, and children! I wanted to have girls, and I wanted to have a son.

And now my son is gone. And I miss him beyond words, my heart hurts, and my stomach aches. I am the unspeakable: a father who has lost a child.

But there are three reasons that I know in my heart of hearts I will find joy again.

1. **Work**. I am going to consciously seek out joy. That

means working on me. It won't be easy or a quick fix, but just like most things in life . . . if you work hard enough on something, you will find success. So, what does that mean? It means continuing to work on my faith. I also desperately want to have peace of mind about where Luke is, as opposed to where he isn't. I believe that joy will come when my family comes together to work through our grief, instead of isolating ourselves.

2. **Legacy.** I am keeping Luke's legacy alive with Team Luke Hope for Minds. Giving hope to others gives me hope and happiness; helping others helps me feel better. By working on remembering his life and fight, I can assist other families and children and provide a fulfilling life for those around me.

3. **God.** I do believe that without my faith in God, I can't find joy amid my pain. I also feel that trying to find joy gives me a purpose. I looked up two verses that I found apply to my mission of finding joy. First Peter 2:19: "For it is commendable if someone bears up under the pain of unjust suffering, because they are conscious of God." And Romans 5:3–4, "We can rejoice, too, when we run into problems and trials, for we know they help us develop endurance. And endurance develops strength of character, and character strengthens our confident hope of salvation."

For you to move on from a difficult or traumatic situation, you have to learn to forgive. For me, the forgiveness aspect of faith is absolutely necessary if I want to find joy again. I am aware of this, but it has been one of my greatest challenges. However, in order for me to really turn the corner on my healing, I must fully commit to forgiving. Not half-way, not some of the time, and not only when I'm in the right frame of mind.

A work in progress for the last seven years, but I will get there. My family deserves it.

"Be kind and compassionate to one another, forgiving each other, just as God forgave you."
— Ephesians 4:32

June 11

Triggers.

I used to be triggered by a baseball field, a school, seeing a golf cart, or watching football. Now breathing is a trigger. All day, every day . . .

Today was no exception. I drove to a middle school to walk on the track, and at a red light I sat for a minute as a funeral procession drove by. I was reminded of August 28, as we drove to Resthaven.

When I got to the track, I put on Bruce Springsteen's most recent album. First song was "One Minute You're Here." The words, "One minute you're here, the next minute you're gone . . ." were a painful reminder of what my family had lost.

Next song was "I'll See You in My Dreams." The lyrics, "I'll see you in my dreams, for death is not the end, and I'll see you in

---

my dreams . . ." had the same effect.

Eventually, a father and son walked to the field and began playing catch. The boy was probably 15 or 16. As I walked around the track, I pictured 16-year-old Luke throwing a ball right at my glove. My favorite thing in the world was to play catch with my son. The fact that I never would again was yet another blow.

I'm not sure if there is a quote more appropriate for me than this:

"Sometimes you have to let go of the picture of what you thought life would be like and learn to find joy in the story you are actually living."

True. And hard.

- Tim

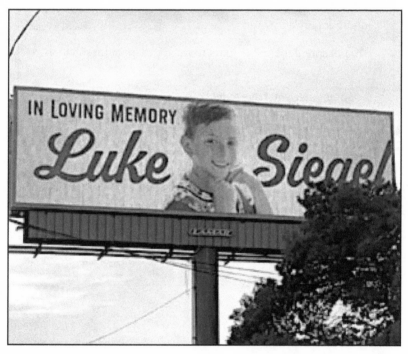

In Loving Memory of Luke Siegel billboard

22

BASEBALL IN HEAVEN

*"Perhaps the only true comfort is
believing I will see you again."*
— Unknown[21]

You may need to sit down when reading this story. This was told to me by Darcy Marshall.

Ty Marshall has Down syndrome. Everyone knew Ty and his good friend, Hannah. She was just a few rooms down the hall from Luke. Hannah was a wonderful girl with an infectious personality who also happened to have Down syndrome. Unfortunately, Hannah passed away a few days after Luke's accident. Hannah was in the ICU just a few doors down from Luke. She will never be forgotten.

Ty suffered a stroke June 16, 2021, and came to Trust-point to do rehab shortly after. At that point, Luke had been going there to do PT three days a week for two years. Trust-point is a wonderful in-patient/out-patient rehab facility where we were blessed to have the most incredible physical therapist, Emily.

On July 1, Ty's mom sent me a message asking me if I would visit Ty while he was outside. I left Luke in the gym with our nurse and walked outside to visit with Darcy and Ty. We chatted for a few minutes about Ty and Luke before I went back inside.

But the danger wasn't over. On September 28, Ty had a nine-hour surgery on his brain. The doctor told Darcy that there was a chance that Ty wouldn't recognize his mom.

Darcy waited and waited anxiously. Finally, she went to see Ty. Immediately he began to speak. "Mom I've been crying for you," he said.

Darcy was so relieved. He knew her. Then the words kept coming, which was uncharacteristic of Ty.

"Mom, I saw Hannah singing and dancing. And I saw Luke Siegel with a baseball in his hand." Darcy was shocked by what Ty had just said, but she wanted to hear more. Ty continued, "The three of us walked away to throw the baseball."

Every time I share this story, I get chills. Most of the time, the person hearing this also gets chills. Why? Because Ty Marshall had never met Luke. He had seen him from a distance in the gym but had never talked to him. Ty never knew that Luke played baseball!

This story is both unbelievable and believable. Was this a near-death experience for Ty? God telling me that Luke was OK?

For me, this is a story that I hold onto every day. And every night. And forever.

For six years, I woke up with the same mindset. Maybe today would be the day that Luke would say his first word.

Every single day I prayed about it and believed with all my heart that Luke would speak.

He had made so much progress. He made sounds that seemed so close to words. I told Luke "I love you" 20 times a day. There was no doubt in my mind that he tried and tried to say it back.

Since the day Luke passed, every morning I wake up with the same mindset. Today Luke will give me a sign that he is doing OK.

My friend Bobby worded it differently. He said that God would give me that sign. Amen.

July 23

A father designed a headstone for his wheelchair-bound son depicting him "free of his earthly burdens."

This picture is certainly worth a thousand words.

This week I spoke to an uncle whose niece fell off the back of a golf cart and suffered a traumatic brain injury.

I visited a young boy in the hospital who was involved in a car accident. I was on the phone with two other parents whose children are recovering from a brain injury.

I saw despair on their faces and heard it in their voices. I ache for them.

Next Thursday will be seven years since Luke's accident. It still seems like yesterday. But the pain feels like a lifetime.

Team Luke Hope for Minds has granted over $500,000 this year. Think about how many families are feeling like their

---

lives have been turned upside down. I pray that they never give up hope.

Take a moment and count your blessings.

- Tim

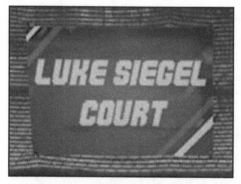

Luke Siegel Court sign

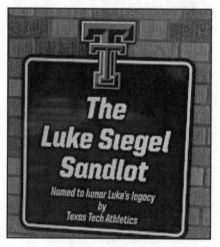

The Luke Siegel Sandlot sign

23

FAMILY FRIDAY

*"Hope. If you only carry one thing throughout your entire
life, let it be hope. Let it be hope that better things are always
ahead. Let it be hope that you can get through even the
toughest of times. Let it be hope that you are stronger than
any challenge that comes your way. Let it be hope that you
are exactly where you are meant to be right now, and that
you are on the path to where you are meant to be... Because
during these times, hope will be the very thing that carries you
through."*
— Unknown[22]

Team Luke Hope for Minds has a very strong social media presence. Here's what we focus on each day of the
week:

Monday—Motivational Monday
Tuesday—Tuesdays with Tim
Wednesday—Wear it Wednesday
Thursday—Thankful Thursday
Friday—Family Friday

Saturday—Safety Saturday

Sunday—Scripture Sunday

On Friday we highlight a family we have helped; this is one of my favorite days. These are a few of their stories:

ELLIE

She was diagnosed with a brain injury in 2019. Her family reached out for assistance in funding treatment at the NAPA Center.

"We cannot begin to thank Team Luke Hope for Minds enough," her mother said. "Ellie made so much progress in this three-week intensive program. Ever since, Ellie has been happier, she is able to move around better, and is actually reaching for her toys.

"Thank you so much for being a major steppingstone in Ellie's journey. Christmas 2021 was one for the books!"

LEVI

Levi was almost three years old when he and his twin brother were in a drowning incident in 2019. Levi suffers from an anoxic brain injury due to a lack of oxygen. His motor functions are gone; he lost the ability to speak, eat by mouth, walk, and so many more functions.

"Team Luke Hope for Minds has helped Levi in so many ways from emotional support to financial support," says Levi's mother, Demi. "Team Luke Hope for Minds helped Levi receive hyperbaric oxygen treatments and helped us with the deposit on an apartment so we can have a place to live. We are forever grateful for TLHFM! The pictures featured are him in his gait trainer and stander! He is learning how to walk and how to do weight-bear again!"

OLIVE

Olive suffered a brain injury from a non-fatal drowning in June 2020. Her family reached out to us in hopes of receiving funds for MNRI treatments.

"Thank you, Team Luke Hope for Minds, for funding Olive's treatments! The day our sweet girl survived a drowning is a day I will never forget. Thankfully she has hope to walk again someday because of the funding for her therapies," her mother Tamara said.

GABBY

She suffered an anoxic brain injury from a non-fatal drowning. Her family reached out to Team Luke Hope for Minds for help in purchasing a medical van to better transport Gabby.

"It started taking a toll on me physically to carry her to the car, and she was so uncomfortable and agitated during car rides," her mother said. "Now that we have a medical van, she has become a whole new person. Car rides are more relaxing since she is sitting comfortably in her special molded wheelchair. She now has more room and head support.

"Taking Gabby to appointments and therapies has become less stressful for her and myself. Thank you so much for your help. God is good."

LUKE

Luke suffered a traumatic brain injury in a boating accident at age six, leaving him non-verbal and immobile.

"We started Hyperbaric Oxygen Therapy after connecting with TLHFM, and within a week Luke began smiling and laughing at jokes," Luke's mother Katie said.

Luke and his family attended our Making Connections in October and connected with Dr. Proefrock. They applied for his stem cell treatments and thanks to our donors, we were able to provide the funds. Recent studies have found that exogenous stem cells can migrate to damaged brain tissue, then participate in the repair of damaged brain tissue by further differentiation to replace damaged cells.

"We are so appreciative of Team Luke Hope for Minds' generous financial support and knowledge provided at the most difficult time in our lives," Katie said.

EZRA

He suffered a loss of oxygen and blood flow to the brain shortly after birth, causing an anoxic brain injury. His family reached out to Team Luke Hope for Minds for assistance in purchasing a hyperbaric oxygen chamber.

"Ezra saw so many improvements while doing HBOT with Dr. Harch," his father said. "Team Luke's support is giving us the opportunity to continue hyperbaric treatment with Ezra at home! This could change the rate of Ezra's progress and improve the quality of his life. This means more than we could ever say to us, and most importantly, to Ezra!"

JOSHUA

After nearly drowning in a kayaking accident in May 2020, Joshua suffered a brain injury. His family reached out to Team Luke Hope for Minds seeking funds for treatment at the Austin Center for Developing Minds. "Since starting with them, our son, who we were told shouldn't be alive and wouldn't regain 'quality of life,' has written his name again, stood again, and regained so many more abilities we were told he'd never have again," his mother Monica said. "Team Luke gave Joshua and our family a chance to live life to the fullest again. God bless Team Luke. Thank you for changing Joshua's life and ours."

MARLEE

At 22 months old, she suffered a brain injury due to a stroke following her third open heart surgery in July 2018. Her family reached out to Team Luke Hope for Minds to help fund hyperbaric oxygen treatments.

"The assistance Team Luke Hope for Minds is giving us will be a life changer for Marlee," her mother said. "It will open up new treatment for her brain injury and allow her to walk and talk in a more fluent manner. We are very grateful for this opportunity. Thank you so much."

STRYKER

On April 21, Stryker suffered a traumatic brain injury when he fell out of a second-story window in his home due to an improper installation. He was in the hospital for a week, and then was closely monitored at home for an additional week.

"Team Luke Hope for Minds reached out to us while we were in the hospital and let us know they were here for us in any way possible," says Stryker's mother, Jessica. "Because of Team Luke Hope for Minds, we were able to pay our rent without having to worry about how we would make it till the next paycheck. We never would have known there was help for us if Team Luke Hope for Minds didn't reach out to us. To know we are not alone during this hard time was such a blessing. We couldn't be more thankful, and we truly appreciate everything they have done for us."

CAMILA

Camila was in a car accident that resulted in many injuries including a spinal cord and traumatic brain injury. The Patino family was in the hospital for nearly six months during her recovery.

"I just want to say that we are very thankful for TLH-FM helping with funds to build a new room and an accessible bathroom for Camila. We are very blessed," Camila's mother, Maria, said. "Having a bigger and more accessible room was something that she needed in order to be more independent. Team Luke Hope for Minds was there for us when we needed them and continues to offer support to us. We cannot thank TLHFM enough."

BEN

He suffered an anoxic brain injury after a non-fatal drowning accident in July 2021. We were able to help his family purchase a hyperbaric oxygen chamber for home use.

"Thank you, Team Luke Hope for Minds, for your assistance," Ben's mother said. "We have seen so many improvements with hyperbaric oxygen treatments and are thrilled to be able to continue this therapy at home with Ben."

NORA

Nora is deaf, blind, and non-mobile/non-verbal. She survived complete heart and respiratory failure, but unfortunately suffered an anoxic brain injury in the process.

"We would like to thank TLHFM for helping us through some of our hard times," Norah's mom, Tabitha, said. "We felt incredibly BLESSED to be able to purchase her new corrective lenses and adaptive equipment that will help her to grow and thrive. When no one else was there, TLHFM was. Thank you for loving us."

SEAN

He was born with a rare defect in his brain and at the age of two, he had an onset of seizures. Unfortunately, the uncontrolled seizures were injuring his brain and he was then clinically diagnosed with cerebral palsy. Sean's conditions have impacted him in many ways in his 14 years.

"Sean is determined and faces obstacles with a smile," Sean's mother, Ruth, said. "Sean attends therapies, doctor appointments, school, and community events. Recently, our family van used to transport Sean in his wheelchair stopped working and was falling apart. Without a van, this would have made things very challenging, and we would not be able to transport Sean safely in his wheelchair. With assistance from Team Luke Hope for Minds, I was able to come up with a down payment so we could finance a new van for Sean. We are grateful and know that everyone is placed in our lives at just the right time. Thank you for being a part of Sean's journey."

ELIZABETH

Elizabeth suffered an anoxic brain injury on May 31, 2021.

"We are so grateful for Team Luke Hope for Minds, it has been a great organization to connect with for our family" Elizabeth's mother, Danielle, said. "It has helped us to receive hyperbaric oxygen therapy, which is only adding to her healing and wholeness. God bless TLHFM!"

SETH

At nine months, Seth was diagnosed with Shaken Baby Syndrome and a Traumatic Brain Injury after being violently shaken and hit in the head by his sitter. He has experienced bad seizures his whole life. Seth is now 16 and cannot be left alone. TLHFM is funding service dog training, which will teach the dog to alert someone if Seth has a seizure, providing Seth with more freedom and independence.

"The help that we have received from Team Luke Hope for Minds is literally a life saver," said Seth's mother, Valerie. "This will give everyone that loves Seth a little peace of mind. I can't begin to thank everyone enough!"

RUBY

Ruby is a brain tumor survivor with a traumatic brain injury as a result of the treatment used to remove the tumor from her cerebellum. Ruby has been cancer-free for three years; however, it left her with ataxia, hypotonia, and general movement impairments that require many hours at rehab and a myriad of other medical expenses.

"We are so grateful for Team Luke Hope for Minds," says Ruby's mother, Jessie. "When insurance refused to cover the physical therapy clinic that we found gave Ruby the best support, TLHFM quickly stepped in to help us. Where insurance has drained us with its conflicting information, piles of confusing paperwork, and no's, working with TLHFM was a breath of fresh air. The application was straightforward, Ronda was so kind when I called with questions, and the 'Yes' to our request was given joyfully. With Team Luke Hope for Minds' help, we have been able to significantly cut the cost of our medical expenses and continue to pursue safety and healing for Ruby. Thank you!"

***

These are just some families that we've helped on their healing journey. We hope to help many more. Through the first half of 2021, we have granted over $500,000 and are receiving applications almost every day. Our team is so honored to help families from all over the country.

When I read these messages from parents, it warms my heart. I understand their pain, but I also know their needs, their questions, and their fear. I feel blessed that we are able to give parents hope and comfort through our organization. We help financially, but I am certain that parents want to feel that their child is given every opportunity to improve. This is every bit as important as the money we provide. We let them know that they are not alone. We are here for them every day. And that makes me proud.

March 29

I was recently asked, what is your WHY?

My job is to help families all over the country: families who are overwhelmed, and families who have no idea if there will be improvements for their child.

Every day when I talk to a parent, or when I speak daily with my staff, I am reminded of what happened to Luke. But I know what my "why" is.

WHAT YOU ARE ABOUT TO READ CONFIRMS WHY I DO WHAT I DO.

> Hi Mr. Siegel. My name is Kellie Burkhart. My son, Andrew, was just blessed with a grant from your amazing organization. I wanted to reach out and say THANK YOU to you and everyone at TLHFM! Your blessing for Andrew is a literal answer to many prayers and we are deeply grateful. We have been on this path of paying all out of pocket for Andrew's medical care for over 12 years now and some days it is very difficult to see how we are going to pay for Andrew's medical treatments moving forward. We have been praying about this frequently for

sure. When we got the email saying Andrew was approved we were at the park and I started crying. I read the email to Andrew and my husband and we all hugged and said "Thank you, Jesus!" right there in the middle of the OR. I just wanted to give you a picture of what your emails look like on the other side. Thank you for giving us a life raft in our effort to help our son heal further.

I have been following Luke's journey and your journey as a family for a couple of years now. I am deeply sorry for your incredible earthly loss of your beautiful boy. I am so inspired by all that you do to help others in the midst of all that you and your family have been and continue to go through. I have and will continue to pray for you all. The transparency with which you share your journey is also very inspiring and helpful to many more people than you will ever know.

Here is a picture of Andrew with a thank you message.

I hope that I get to meet you someday so that I can thank you in person. God bless you all!

—Kellie

I look forward to taking Kellie and her family to an Arizona Cardinals game this fall.

This message from Kellie gives me strength and a purpose to put one foot in front of the other.

- Tim

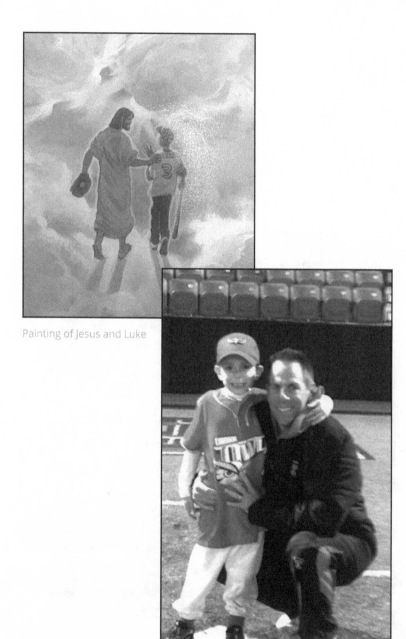

Painting of Jesus and Luke

Luke and Tim on baseball field

24

MY HEAD ON THE PILLOW

"When you awaken in the morning's hush
I am the swift uplifting rush
Of quiet birds in circled flight.
I am the soft stars that shine at night.
Do not stand at my grave and cry;
I am not there; I did not die."
— Mary Elizabeth Frye[23]

Every single night since Luke passed, my bedtime routine has remained the same.

I take Trazadone, a slow-acting, long-lasting sleeping pill. I then lay my head on the pillow, take three deep breaths, and talk to God.

I try not to think about Luke. A few seconds later, I think about Luke. Occasionally, these thoughts are from Luke's first nine years. The happy times, the healthy times, and the times we talked and played sports. A precious memory of Luke in the dugout or dropping Luke off for school and knowing just a second or two later, he would turn around and wave. Or when we threw the football in the front yard, pretending to be the New Orleans Saints. I focused on the days Luke had sleepovers, or those times Luke yelled at me to watch him play Madden football. He loved to show me the score of his Saints destroying the Dallas Cowboys.

But those sweet, happy memories don't last long. Unfortunately, sadness, disbelief, anger, and helplessness take over.

I toss and turn, trying desperately to turn my attention to something else. My to-do list for the next day might distract me for a minute or two. The mom or dad I just talked to might occupy my brain. Then I might imagine what they were going through at that very moment. And then back to Luke.

My best distraction is the worst thing for sleep: my cell phone. I tell myself, don't grab it. Nine times out of ten, I pick it up and look to see the results I might have missed on ESPN. Twitter works as a distraction. I check email and some text messages.

Every once in a while, I look at videos and pictures. This is like sticking myself with a needle.

The videos I took of Jersey and Olive, our incredible golden doodles, make me smile, but then the picture of Luke at therapy or the one of us in the chair make my stomach ache.

Eventually, the Trazadone puts me to sleep.

Then I wake up in the middle of the night: two, three, or four, nearly every morning, without fail. Sometimes, I have to go to the bathroom and sometimes there is no reason at all.

For six years, I either woke up with Luke in the middle of the night, or I woke up to check on Luke, so maybe my brain was used to this crazy schedule.

Ten months later, nothing has made a difference. God, I wish this pattern would change.

I'm well aware of what not to do when it applies to good sleep. Stay off the phone, keep the TV off, don't turn the lights on, stay away from the pantry, etc., etc., etc.

That advice doesn't apply to a father who lost his son, his hero, his little buddy.

Isn't it fitting that I'm yawning as I write these words?

My health is my top priority, and good sleep is vitally important to keeping me healthy.

I'll get there, hopefully sooner rather than later. Tonight, when you put your head on your pillow, be thankful that you haven't lost a child. Or if you have lost a child, talk to a doctor about the best medicine for sleep. And if you are like millions of people who struggle to sleep because of your job, your kids, your personal life, or all of the above, I hope that you find something that works for you.

I pray that tonight as I put my head on the pillow, I will think less and sleep more.

July 20

I think about him when I talk to parents.

I think about him when I see a baseball field.

I think about him when I see a school.

I think about him when I see the number 3.

I think about him when I see his friends.

I think about him when I'm at church.

I think about him when I walk.

I think about him when watch sports on TV.

I think about him when I lay my head on the pillow.

- Tim

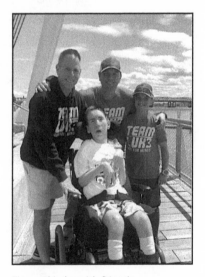

Tim and Luke with friends

25

KEEPING LUKE'S LEGACY ALIVE

"Hope is important because it can make the present moment less difficult to bear. If we believe that tomorrow will be better, we can bear a hardship today."
— Thich Nhat Hanh[24]

Remembering and honoring Luke will be my mission until I take my last breath.

I have heard many comments since Luke passed.

"Luke is in a better place."

"Luke is healed."

"Luke isn't suffering anymore."

"Luke is playing baseball in heaven."

"Luke is so proud of you."

"Luke's legacy will live forever."

The last quote is the one that motivates me for so many reasons. I believe the others to be true, but the one about keeping Luke's legacy alive keeps me alive.

I don't want anyone to forget Luke. I want people to remember his fight and his determination. And before the accident, his sweet disposition and his thoughtfulness of others.

Luke was such an inspiration and will be forever. He motivated me and is a source of motivation to thousands and thousands, across the world.

But people are busy with their lives, their families, and their jobs. Therefore, it is easy to forget. I will do my best to remind people, in case they do. I hope that sharing our story on social media and continuing to speak to schools, teams, and businesses will keep Luke alive in your heart.

Number 3. This number is associated with Luke all over Lubbock, Texas, and beyond. Jenny and I grew up loving #3, and then Luke took it to another level. Almost every day, I receive a text from a mom or a dad showing me their child's new soccer or baseball number. Kids are asking their coaches if they can wear number 3 in loving memory of Luke.

The Team Luke Hope for Minds shirts are a perfect reminder. We turned the E to a 3 on all our shirts, so they read "LUK3." It seems that every day I spot someone wearing a Team LUK3 shirt. And almost every time I am asked to take a picture with a team, someone in the group suggests that we hold up three fingers to honor Luke.

I've read where the number 3 is considered to be the perfect number, the number of harmonies, wisdom, and understanding. It was also the number of time—past, present, and future; birth, life, and death; beginning, middle, end—the number of the divine.

The number 3 appears in the Bible 467 times. Of course, we can't look at the number 3 without looking at the

Trinity: the Father, Son, and Holy Spirit. The number 3 carries an extreme significance throughout scripture. It's either pointing to the importance of something or showing the completeness of something. So, when you see the number 3, think of Luke, and when you do, think of 3 words.

Fight Like Luke.

These are the 3 most important words for me. I remind others to fight like Luke while I'm reminding myself to do the same. Luke's strength gave me strength and will do so for the rest of my life.

"Fight Like Luke" has taken a life of its own. Teams, schools, and friends use this as their motto. Luke was the greatest fighter I have ever seen. For 6 years under the direst circumstances, Luke never gave up. His fighting spirit lives on forever.

Team Luke Hope for Minds will definitely keep Luke's legacy alive. Every family we help will forever be linked to Luke. Because of Luke's accident, hundreds of families are benefitting financially, educationally, and emotionally.

This doesn't take the pain away, but it does give me comfort. Luke's impact, along with Team Luke Hope for Minds, will continue for many generations to come.

Luke was the perfect son. I waited 42 years before I had him, and he was worth the wait: my hero, my buddy.

Luke, you are in my heart, every waking moment. I love you so much. You have branded my heart; on and under my skin.

<u>7 YEARS AGO . . .</u>

On July 28, 2015, Luke was in a golf cart accident.

Time heals? Not when it comes to this day. Seven years later and I find myself going over everything leading up to the second that I got that phone call . . . "I think Luke broke his nose."

To the moment I arrived at the scene of the accident.

To pacing the halls whispering the same thing I said to Luke every single day. "You're my boy."

To the words, "Luke was in cardiac arrest for 7 minutes."

To all of our friends in the waiting room.

To praying to God that Luke would make it . . .

As much as I love #3, I absolutely cringe when I see #28.

The pain is still so real, 7 years later.

I was in Atlanta this week, hoping to raise awareness and funds for TLHFM. I was having lunch with a special woman named Arlene when she said something to me that stopped me in my tracks.

"You are turning PAIN into PASSION."

So simple, yet so profound.

Today is a very, very hard day for our family. They all are, but this one takes me to a place that shatters my heart in tiny little pieces . . . all over again. This was the worst day of our lives. For Jenny, and Luke's sisters.

I want to thank you for your support, your prayers, your messages, and your encouragement over these last 7 years.

Luke's accident should never have happened. But anger, rage, frustration, sadness, and fear have slowly moved to hope, strength, forgiveness, and faith.

And when I am down like I am today, I will always remember what Arlene told me.

I'm turning pain into passion.

My passion to help other families will be my calling until I take my last breath.

- Tim

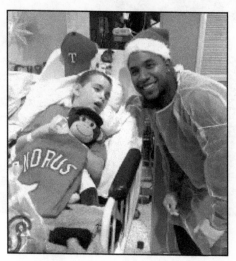

Luke and Elvis Andrus

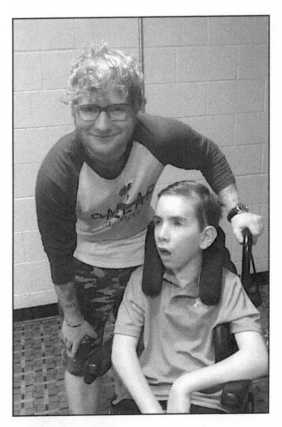

Luke and Ed Sheeran

26

MY DREAMS

"Why you died, I will never understand; but I have a million reasons why you lived."
— Andy Weir[25]

I dream every night, and they are always so vivid. I've always felt that they were telling me something. Sure, some were random, but many seemed to hit me right in the heart.

Believe it or not, I still have dreams about coaching tennis.

After Luke's accident, my dreams were always the same: I was in the kitchen with one of the girls when suddenly Luke began to speak. This happened just a few times, but always the same dream. Maybe that is why I was so sure that Luke would eventually talk.

I've had three very real and meaningful dreams since Luke passed.

The first dream: On September 15, I dreamt that I was just behind Luke while he was in his wheelchair. He was in therapy. Three therapists were in front of him. He began waving his hands as if to say, "Goodbye, I don't need you anymore."

The second dream: I was driving Jenny's grandmother to her speaking engagement. But there were dead ends everywhere I turned. Finally, I found my way out. When we arrived, I was told that the speech was to be given by me. The audience was to both my left and right. For some reason, nobody was directly in front of me. As I began to share my inspirations from Luke, I stopped and told the crowd that I was going to get Luke. I brought him right in front of me. Then suddenly, Luke got out of his wheelchair and got on a bike and rode it back and forth.

The third dream: I was walking Luke in his wheelchair. We were shopping. We stopped to get a waffle. Someone told me that Luke wasn't alive, even though I was pushing him. I said it's OK, he is here with me now.

I've always been someone who likes to analyze dreams, mine especially. They resonate with me in a profound way. I'm being told something by someone: that is how I see it.

Some would find this thinking out in left field, but I choose to believe that they hit home. These three dreams are no coincidence. Some random person asking me why I am still pushing Luke in his wheelchair if he isn't alive. He is alive—in my heart and in my soul.

Luke in front of three therapists and waving his arms goodbye. He couldn't move his arms, but in his dream, he was saying thank you and goodbye.

The fact that there were no chairs right in front of my speech, when I suddenly decided to bring Luke out of his room. I put him in the middle and shockingly he crawls to his bike and rides it back and forth. Luke and I rode bikes almost every day when he was seven, eight, and nine years old.

These were dreams, but they were much more than that to me.

**

How often does our life fall exactly as planned?

I loved tennis and I wanted to be a professional. My dream as a kid was to play at Wimbledon and compete against the best in the world. It happened. But that happened because of hard work, dedication, and determination.

Did I plan to coach tennis at Texas Tech when I had just finished professional tennis? No, I didn't. Did I ever plan to go from college coaching to high school and middle school coaching? Never in a million years.

Did I ever think I would be the executive director of a nonprofit? I didn't know the first thing about a nonprofit.

Did I ever think that my little baseball player would have suffered a brain injury and then pass away at the tender age of 15?

But what I do think is that I am on this earth to make a difference and to keep Luke's legacy alive. And I will do this until I take my last breath.

June 29

The little things . . .

I was looking though old pictures tonight and decided to share pictures of Luke before the accident.

And then I thought of something.

The little things we did together were not little. As a matter of fact, nothing you do with your child is little. Playing cards with Luke, taking the kids to a TTU baseball game, watching the Saints game . . . all big things I never took for granted. We took the kids on vacations, to professional sporting events, and travelled with them to their games.

Those were big things.

But what I really miss with Luke are the simple little things. Just talking, watching TV, playing catch, going to get ice cream, and eating dinner with the whole family.

Don't ever take those times for granted.

One thing is certain . . . doing those "little" things will continue with my girls and my grandsons.

One foot in front of the other.

- Tim

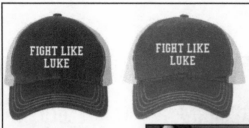

Fight Like Luke hats

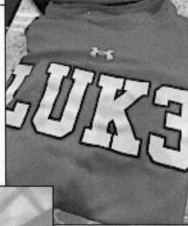

Luk3 t-shirt

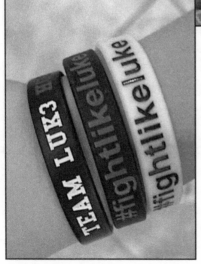

TLHFM wristbands

Congressional Record

United States of America

PROCEEDINGS AND DEBATES OF THE 117th CONGRESS, FIRST SESSION

WASHINGTON, TUESDAY, OCTOBER 26, 2021

House of Representatives

RECOGNIZING THE LIFE OF LUKE SIEGEL

HON. JODEY C. ARRINGTON
OF TEXAS
IN THE HOUSE OF REPRESENTATIVES
Tuesday, October 26, 2021

Mr. ARRINGTON. Madam Speaker, I rise today to recognize the life of a remarkable young man named Luke Siegel, who inspired so many with his strength of spirit and will to live in the face of tremendous adversity.

On July 28 of 2015, Luke suffered severe brain damage as a result of a tragic golf cart accident that changed his life forever and left him immobile, lifeless, and even without the ability to speak. Doctors said, Madam Speaker, that he would stay in that condition as long as he lived.

But, through the love and support of his family, the prayers of our wonderful community, and the relentless and tenacious fight that Luke brought every day, he defied all odds and the diagnoses of numerous doctors, recovering to a life no one believed was possible.

Sadly, on August 19, our hero and west Texas warrior, Luke Siegel, went home to be with his Heavenly Father. Luke is survived by one amazing family: father, Tim; mother, Jenny; and sisters Alex, Kate, and Ellie.

Madam Speaker, Luke never gave up. He was a symbol of hope for people throughout the country whose families have struggled with the challenges of traumatic brain injury. Luke is an inspiration to us all to live every day to the fullest and never give up no matter what the circumstances.

I am confident that Luke Siegel heard those beautiful and sweet words of our creator and Lord of heaven and Earth.

Madam Speaker, Luke fought the good fight, he finished the race, and he kept the faith. May Luke enter into his eternal rest.

God bless Luke Siegel, coach, your family, and God bless west Texas.

God bless the Siegel family. Love & respect, Jodey

Congressional Record recognizing the life of Luke Siegel

ACKNOWLEDGMENTS

To God for giving me the strength to put one foot in front of the other.

To Ronda Johnson, my partner with Team Luke Hope for Minds—you are the hardest worker I know.

To Chuck Angel, pastor of Turning Point Community Church. Our time together has helped more than you know.

To Andre Agassi for your continued support.

To Chelsea Sims, my incredible assistant.

To all of Luke's doctors, nurses, and therapists. Thank you for all you do.

To Kliff Kingsbury for your continued support.

To Andy Roddick, John Isner, and Luke Jensen—thank you for all you have meant to Team Luke Hope for Minds.

To Bruce Springsteen—your music is my therapy.

To Dick Vitale for your support.

To Patricia Jensen for all you do for our mission.

To Lubbock, Texas and the Texas Tech Athletic department for your unwavering support.

To Drew Brees for being the best hero a little boy could have.

To Patrick Mahomes for always wearing the Team Luke Hope for Minds bracelet on your right wrist.

To Mark Styslinger—without your support, Team Luke Hope for Minds wouldn't be where we are today.

To my staff and board at Team Luke Hope for Minds for your hard work and dedication.

To everyone all over the world for your thoughts and prayers.

To Lauren Hall, Whitney Gossett, and your team at Content Capital.

To Bobby Banck—the best friend a guy could ever have.

To my close friends who have been there for me these last seven years.

To Jenny and my girls, Alex, Kate, and Ellie. I love you all so much.

To Luke . . . my hero. My inspiration. You are in my heart every minute of every day.

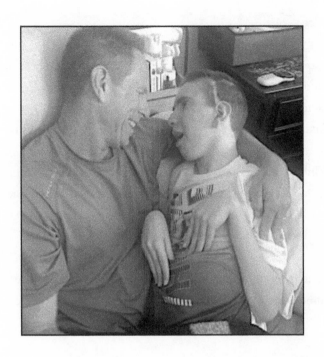

ABOUT THE AUTHOR

Tim Siegel has been passionate about sports his whole life. He is a former professional tennis player and has competed in all four Grand Slam events. From 1993–2015, he was a much-respected tennis coach at Texas Tech University and won Big 12 Coach of the Year two times. He has also led two doubles teams to the finals of the NCAA Championships.

In 2019, Tim was inducted into the Arkansas Razorback Hall of Fame and in 2022 into the Louisiana Tennis Hall of Fame.

His accomplishments after 2015 were not strictly focused on his tennis career, but have brought even more value and purpose to his life. In 2019 he wrote *It's in God's Hands*, a heartfelt memoir about surviving and coping with his son's traumatic brain injury, and is currently the executive director of Team Luke Hope for Minds, a nonprofit that supports children throughout the world after brain injury. He hopes to make the world safer for children and provide families with resources to navigate the difficult journey of recovery and rehabilitation.

A proud father and grandfather, he has three lovely daughters, three beautiful grandsons, and a granddaughter on the way.

NOTES

1. "Susan Zola LCSW Therapist Long Island New York." Words of Wisdom | Susan Zola Licensed Social Worker. Accessed August 12, 2022. https://www.susanzola.com/resources/words-of-wisdom/.

2. Lynn, Larry. "Inspirational Quote for 1.29.15: Grieving for Her Daughter." AfterTalk, January 22, 2015. https://blog.aftertalk.com/inspirational-quote-1-29-15-grieving-daughter/.

3. Troy, Gemma. "Free Gemma Troy - I Miss You in Ways That Not Even Words Can Understand. - JPG." Template.net. Accessed August 12, 2022. https://www.template.net/editable/102526/gemma-troy-i-miss-you-quotes.

4. Kane, Toni. "I Miss You So Much." Greeting Cards for Facebook, January 7, 2020. https://www.all-greatquotes.com/if-people-knew-how-much-i-truly-missed-you/.

5. Kane, Toni. "We Were Blessed to Have You." Greeting Cards for Facebook, July 19, 2021. https://www.all-greatquotes.com/in-these-moment-of-heartbreaking-grief-quote/.

6. Jurski, Kris. "Don't Ask God Why He's Allowing Something to Happen. Ask Him What He Wants You to Learn and Do in the Midst of It.: Inspired to Reality." Inspired to Reality | Motivational Quotes and Stories, April 11, 2016. https://www.inspiredtoreality.com/pin/dont-ask-god-why-hes-allowing-something-to-happen-ask-him-what-he-wants-you-to-learn-and-do-in-the-midst-of-it/.

7. Kane, Toni. "Grief Is Like Having Broken Ribs." Greeting Cards for Facebook, April 11, 2022. https://www.all-greatquotes.com/grief-is-like-having-broken-ribs/.

8. Morris, Pam. "Broken Things Can Become Blessed Things If You Let God Do the Mending!" HubPages. HubPages, July 11, 2022. https://discover.hubpages.com/religion-philosophy/httppammorrishubpagescomhubBroken-things-can-become-Blessed-things-if-we-let-God-do-the-Mending.

9. Daily Inspirational Quotes. "The Storm That Was Sent to Break You, Is Going to Be the Storm..." Daily Inspirational Quotes, March 23, 2018. https://www.dailyinspirationalquotes.in/2018/03/

the-storm-that-was-sent-to-break-you-is-going-to-be-the-storm-that-god-uses-to-make-you/.

10. Kane, Toni. "You Are Always in My Heart." Greeting Cards for Facebook, June 15, 2022. https://www.all-greatquotes.com/time-passes-but-not-one-day-goes-by-grief-quote/.

11. Cacciatore, Joanne. "If You Simply Cannot Understand Why Someone Is Grieving So Much, for So Long, Then Consider Yourself Fortunate That You Do Not Understand. – Joanne Cacciatore Https://T.co/6hyyr20dea." Twitter. Twitter, December 8, 2019. https://twitter.com/dr_cacciatore/status/1203722336970526720?lang=en.

12. "Today, You Could Be Standing next to Someone Who Is Doing All They Can to Not Fall Apart..: Meaningful Quotes, Wise Quotes, Quotable Quotes." Pinterest, June 30, 2020. https://www.pinterest.com/pin/today-you-could-be-stand-ing-next-to-someone-who-is-doing-all-they-can-to-not-fall-apart--529595237436202622/.

13. Lusko, Levi. "Pain Is a Microphone." FaithGateway Store. Accessed August 12, 2022. https://faithgateway.com/blogs/christian-books/pain-is-a-microphone.

14. Castaneda, Clearissa Lynn. "Choose to Keep Going." Medium. Medium, April 28, 2019. https://medium.com/@clearissalynncas-taneda/choose-to-keep-going-%EF%B8%8F-80204c01f993.

15. MacArthur, Tori. "Memorial Day Quotes about Remembrance." Online Education Courses for Youth and Non Traditional Students Coral Sands Academy, May 23, 2022. https://coralsandsacademy.com/memorial-day-quotes-about-remembrance/.

16. Johnson, Samuel Decker. "A Quote by Samuel Decker Thompson." Goodreads. Goodreads, 2018. https://www.goodreads.com/quotes/9107015-we-are-all-just-a-car-crash-a-diagnosis-an.

17. Beecher, Henry Ward. "Henry Ward Beecher Quotes." Brainy-Quote. Xplore. Accessed August 12, 2022. https://www.brainy-quote.com/quotes/henry_ward_beecher_382348.

18. "64 Quotes after Grief and Life after Loss What's Your Grief." What's your Grief, August 2, 2022. https://whatsyourgrief.com/64-quotes-about-grief/.

19. Li, Lesya. "Finding Balance between Holding on and Letting Go." HavingTime, August 23, 2017. https://havingtime.com/find-ing-balance-holding-letting-go/.

20. "Trust in His Timing Rely on His Promises Wait for His Answers Believe in His Miracles Rejoice in His Goodness Relax in His Presence." Like this poster. Accessed August 12, 2022. https://keepcalms.com/p/trust-in-his-timing-rely-on-his-promises-wait-for-his-answers-believe-in-his-miracles-rejoice-in-his-goodness-re-lax-in-his-presence/.

21. "42 Heartfelt Grief Quotes for Loss." Greeting Cards for Facebook, January 23, 2022. https://www.all-greatquotes.com/grief-quotes/.

22. Daher, Ali. "Bindi Irwin Shares an Insiprational Message of Hope amid Coronavirus Outbreak." Daily Mail Online. Associated Newspapers, March 16, 2020. https://www.dailymail.co.uk/tvshowbiz/article-8118879/Bindi-Irwin-shares-insiprational-mes-sage-hope-amid-coronavirus-outbreak.html.

23. Morrow, Angela. "Inspiring Poems about Death, Grief, and Loss to Help in a Time of Need." Verywell Health. Verywell Health, February 23, 2020. https://www.verywellhealth.com/words-of-in-spiration-1132544.

24. Nhat Hanh, Thich. "A Quote from Peace Is Every Step." Goodreads. Goodreads. Accessed August 12, 2022. https://www.goodreads.com/quotes/124838-hope-is-important-because-it-can-make-the-present-moment.

25. Weir, Andy. The Egg. Accessed August 12, 2022. http://galactanet.com/oneoff/theegg_mod.html.

RESOURCES

To donate to TLHFM:

Teamlukehopeforminds.org

To follow TLHFM on Twitter, Instagram, Facebook:

@teamlukehopeforminds

To follow Tim Siegel:

Facebook: Prayforlukesiegel

Instagram @Luke.Siegel

Twitter. @TimsiegelTTU

9 781954 020405